WALKED OUT OF THE NEW ROAD

— *to* —

CONQUER CANCER

VOLUME III

Walked Out of the New Way of Cancer Treatment
with Immune Regulation and Control of the
Combination of Chinese and Western Medicine

How to overcome cancer? How to treat cancer?

Part II

Authors: Xu Ze (China) ; Xu Jie(China) ; Bin Wu(America)
Translators: Bin Wu ; Lily Xu ; Zihao Xu ; Bo Wu
Editors: Bin Wu ; Lily Xu ; Tao Wu
Illustrators: Lily Xu ; Bin Wu

authorHOUSE®

AuthorHouse™
1663 Liberty Drive
Bloomington, IN 47403
www.authorhouse.com
Phone: 1 (800) 839-8640

Published by AuthorHouse 02/08/2019

ISBN: 978-1-5462-7690-6 (sc)
ISBN: 978-1-5462-7855-9 (e)

Library of Congress Control Number: 2019900645

Print information available on the last page.

WALKED OUT OF THE NEW ROAD

to

CONQUER CANCER

VOLUME III

(XZ-C cancer treatment new idea)

Walked Out of the New Way of Cancer Treatment with Immune Regulation and Control of the Combination of Chinese and Western Medicine

How to overcome cancer? How to treat cancer?

(Part II)

Contents

Introduction to this book xi

The main concept of the book.. xiii

A Brief Introduction to The first Author xv

A Brief Introduction to the Second Author... xvii

A brief introduction to the third author and the main translator and the main editor........... xix

A Brief introduction to the illustrator and the advisor....................................... xxi

Acknowledgements.. xxiii

Foreword xxv

I. Over the past 30 years, it has walked out a new road of cancer treatment with immunomodulation of the combination of Chinese and Western medicine 1

First, the theoretical system of XZ-C immunomodulation and cancer treatment has been formed, and it has been undergoing the clinical application and observation verification.

(1) Concept of cancer treatment..9

(2) Cancer etiology and pathogenesis...13

(3) Theoretical basis and experimental basis for cancer treatment.....................20

(4) Principles of Cancer Treatment..28

(5) Cancer treatment mode..37

(6) Principles of cancer metastasis treatment...44

(7) New concept of cancer metastasis treatment 48

(8) How to stop or prevent cancer metastasis? "three steps" of anti-cancer metastasis treatment 54

(9) Cancer treatment methods and drugs..59

(10) Research on new concepts and new methods of cancer metastasis treatment 77

(11) The formation of the theoretical system of XZ-C immune regulation and treatment of cancer 87

Second, The book proposed the new concept of XZ-C cancer treatment, and analyzed and compared with traditional therapy, using table analysis and using Introduction

II. Innovation must have challenges to traditional concepts and reform can develop.....91

Foreword...93

(1)   *Analysis, evaluation and questioning of systemic intravenous chemotherapy for solid tumors*...101

    • *Analysis and questioning of the route of systemic intravenous chemotherapy for solid tumor*..101
    • *Analysis and questioning on the calculation method of the dose of systemic intravenous chemotherapy for solid tumor*..101
    • *Analysis and evaluation of the efficacy standard of systemic intravenous chemotherapy for solid tumors*..101

(2)   *Retrospect, analysis and review of the three major treatments of cancer tradition*..........110

    • *Through review, analysis and reflection, discover the problems and drawbacks of traditional therapy*..110

(3)   *Chemotherapy needs further research and improvement*.............................124

    • *There are some important misunderstandings in current chemotherapy*..................124
    • *The main contradiction of traditional chemotherapy*.............................124

(4)   *The initiative to change the solid body tumor intravenous chemotherapy into the target organ intravascular chemotherapy*...133

    • *Advocacy for traditional cancer therapies*...133
    • *Assessment of problems and disadvantages of solid body tumor intravenous chemotherapy*...133
    • *To change and perform the Intravascular chemotherapy into the target organ intravenous chemotherapy for solid tumors*...133
    • *The initiative of specific methods and approaches of target organ intravascular chemotherapy of abdominal solid tumor*...133

(5)   *Initiatives to strategies of improving cancer postoperative adjuvant chemotherapy*.........144

    • *Why should cancer postoperative adjuvant chemotherapy be performed ?*.................144
    • *The analysis of reasons why Postoperative chemotherapy did not meet the desired*....144
    • *how to do cancer postoperative adjuvant chemotherapy well*..................144

(6)   *The opinion of improvement and perfection of the traditional chemotherapy cancer treatment*..155

- *Discussion about the "get" and "lost" after the use of anti-cancer drugs*..................155
- *The status of tumor chemotherapy is the main reason for further improvement of efficacy*...155
- *Suggestions for improving and improving chemotherapy* 155

(7)   *the basic model and specific programs of anti-cancer metastasis*................................162

- *The basic pattern of anti-cancer metastasis* 162
- *The specific treatment plansof anti-cancer metastasis*..162
- *Immunotherapy plays an important role in anticancer treatment* 162

(8)   *the new models and new methods of cancer treatment* 168

- *Strengthen immunotherapy, to improve adverse reactions to chemotherapy*.............168
- *Change intermittent treatment for continuous treatment*.......................................168
- *change the damage to the host into protecting the host*..168
- *change the potential of the tumor and the host, and strive imbalance into the balance* 168
- *change from damaging the central immune organs into protecting the central immune organs*...168
- *change the injury therapy into non-injury therapy*..168

(9)   *"Three Steps" of Anti-cancer Metastasis Therapy* 176

- *The metastasis step should be understood so that the goal of treatment is more specific* 176
- *Try to break each step by step* 176
- *Three major strategies of anti-cancer treatment (trilogy)* 176

(10) *Review and Analysis of Clinical Cases of Adjuvant Chemotherapy for Cancer Surgery*.....182

- *The cases of cancer postoperative adjuvant chemotherapy failed to prevent recurrence* 182
- *The cases of cancer postoperative adjuvant chemotherapy failed to prevent metastasis* 182
- *The cases of chemotherapy to promote immune failure*...182

(11) *Review and Prospect of Treatment of Oncology Surgery*..205

- *The achievement of surgical resection of the tumor in the 20th century*...................205
- *21st century surgical goal should be prevention and treatment research for cancer recurrence and metastasis after surgery radical resection* 205
- *The design of tumor radical surgery should be further studied and perfected*...........205

- *The molecular biology basic research and clinical basic research of metastasis should be strengthened after the radical resection*..*205*
- *To prevent cancer recurrence and metastasis should be done from the surgery*..........*205*

III. The Brief and Easy-Reading Epitome of Walking out the New Way of Conquering Cancer 217

Introduction to this book

Bin Wu

Science is endless and only those who are not afraid of danger or difficult work can reach the science peak. Dr. Xu Ze has been working in the cancer therapy for more than 60 years and works very hard day and night to do the basis and clinical oncology science for the patients and for our human being. In this book all of the contents are from his hard work and from his experiments and **from his excellent or superb surgery skills**, in which has two parts: Part I and Part II and three main topics are explained and demonstrated : 1. The reasons and the theoretical foundation of immune therapy, that is, **what is the theoretical basis of immune therapy which all of evidence are from his actual basic and clinical experiments; 2. How to use our immune therapy to treat the cancer patients? 3. Our clinical verification of our immune therapy is successful.** For example, During the animal experiments of making the tumor-bearing animal models, it was found that when Thymus was removed or the immune suppressor was used, the tumor-bearing animal models can be set up; **he found that immune function has close relation to cancer occurrence and metastasis.** During another of the cancer animal experiment, the body immune system can destroy 10^6 cancer cell so that the immune function should be protected and be activated and should be considered during the cancer prevention and treatment, etc, there are many new discoveries during the basic and clinical experiment. The most excellent things during his research are the series of anti-cancer and anti-cancer metastasis products or medications. After many years of difficult research and application of immune therapy together, the new road of cancer treatment have been working out. All of the contents in this book are the results and achievement of Dr. Xu Ze's hard work and his dedications to our human being and all of the contents are his talent scientific thinking and his high wisdom and his hard work day and night. Dr. Xu Ze has high surgery skills such as he made all of the tumor-bearing animal models and set up the animal modes for lymph and blood metastasis animal mode and the animal mode which the relations between hormone(pregnancy animal) and cancer, the animal model with cancer microcirculation and with the cancer new blood vessel formation which the new medications was found for stopping the tumor blood vessel growth, etc. **It needs the meticulous and high surgery skills to finish all of these procedure in the animal and in the human**. The dedication of Dr. Xu Ze is worth for all of us to learn. His oncology research model is based on **patient-centered** to discover question from clinical work, then come back to the in-depth animal experiments, and then turn to the clinical application in order to improve overall level of health care and ultimately the patient gets the benefits. **<u>The innovation brings the improvement and the progression.</u>**

Finally, due to finishing the books in such a short time and there are huge information in the book and day and night hard work, if there is any mistake, please forgive us and look forward to the feedback.

Bin Wu
12-18-2019 in Lutherville, Maryland in America

The main concept of the book

Walked out of the new way of cancer treatment with immune regulation and control of the combination of Chinese and Western medicine

- Strive to take the road of independent innovation with Chinese characteristics, and adhere to the road of independent innovation of the combination of Chinese and Western medicine with "Chinese-style anti-cancer"
- Walked out of the new road of cancer treatment of XZ-C immune regulation and control of the combination of Chinese and Western medicine at the molecular level
- It has formed the theoretical system of treatment of cancer with XZ-C immune regulation and control which provides the theoretical basis and experimental basis for cancer immunotherapy
- The series products and adaptation range of XZ-C immune regulation and control anti-cancer Chinese medication
- XZ-C immunomodulation anticancer Chinese medications are the result of the modernization of traditional Chinese medication

(Part II)

A Brief Introduction to The first Author

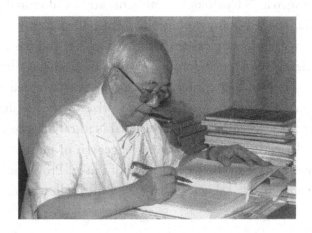

Xu Ze was born in 1933 in Leping City, Jiangxi Province in China. He graduated from Tongji Medical College in 1956. He served as the director of surgery, professor, chief physician, master and doctoral tutor of the Affiliated Hospital of Hubei College of Traditional Chinese Medicine. He is the director of the Experimental Surgery Research Institute of Hubei College of Traditional Chinese Medicine, director of the Department of Abdominal Oncology Surgery, and anti-cancer metastasis, the director of Recurrence Research Office; concurrently serves as executive director of Wuhan Branch of Chinese Medical Association, honorary president of Wuhan Anticancer Research Association, academic member of International Liver Disease Research Collaboration Center, member of International Federation of Surgeons, Chinese Journal of Experimental Surgery No. 1, 2, 3 The 4th Standing Editorial Board and the 1st, 2nd and 3rd Executive Editors of the Journal of Abdominal Surgery. He has been engaged in surgical work for 60 years and has extensive clinical experience in the surgical treatment of lung cancer, esophageal cancer, gastric cancer, liver cancer, gallbladder cancer, pancreatic cancer, and intestinal cancer etc, as well as the combination of Chinese and Western medicine to prevent postoperative recurrence and metastasis. In 1987, he began experimental research on tumors. Through cancer cell transplantation, he established tumor animal models, explored the mechanisms and rules of cancer metastasis and recurrence, and searched for ways to inhibit metastasis and screened 48 kinds of natural drugs from anti-cancer invasion and metastasis and relapsed Chinese medicine, and based on this, he developed xz-c immunomodulation anticancer traditional Chinese medicine preparation, which were clinically verified by a large number of cases and the effect is remarkable. He published 126 scientific research papers and published "New Understanding and New Model of Cancer Treatment", published by Hubei Science and Technology Publishing House and published by Xinhua Bookstore in 2001, In 2006, he published the monograph "New Concept and New Method of Cancer Metastasis Treatment" published by Beijing People's Military Medical Publishing House and published by Xinhua Bookstore. In April 2007, he was awarded the original book award and certificate by the General Administration of Press and Publication of the People's Republic of China. In October 2011, the third monograph (New Concepts and New Methods of Cancer Treatment) was published by Beijing People's Military Medical Press. Xu Ze, Xu Jie/ Zhang, Xinhua Bookstore was released. This book was translated into English by Dr. Bin Wu., published in Washington, DC on March 26, 2013, international distribution. He participated in 10 medical monographs such as "Hepatology Treatment" and "Abdominal Surgery". He engaged in teaching for 60 years, trained many young physicians, 10 master students And 2 doctoral students. He has been engaged in surgical research for 34 years and has achieved many results. Among them, "self-made XZ-C$_1$ type abdominal cavity-venous bypass device for the treatment of cirrhotic refractory ascites and its clinical application" was awarded the Hubei Provincial Government Science and Technology for the second prize of the results, and promoted and applied in 38 hospitals across the country: The National Natural Science Foundation of China's experimental study on the pathophysiology and pathogenesis of pulmonary schistosomiasis by experimental surgical methods won the second prize of Hubei Provincial Government Science and Technology Achievements. He enjoys Special government allowance.

A Brief Introduction to the Second Author

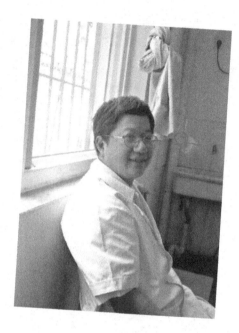

Xu Jie, male, graduated from Hubei College of Traditional Chinese Medicine in 1992, graduated from Hubei Medical University in 1996, Department of Clinical Medicine. Now He is chief physician in Hubei University of Traditional Chinese Medicine Hospital and Hubei Provincial Hospital of Surgery, engaged in experimental surgical tumor research and general surgery, urology clinical work.

Since 1992, he has been involved in the experimental tumor research of the Institute of Experimental Surgery of Hubei College of Traditional Chinese Medicine. He has carried out cancer cell transplantation and established a tumor animal model. He has carried out a series of experimental tumor research: exploring the mechanism of recurrence and metastasis of cancer and in vivo screening experiment of more than 200 kinds of Chinese herbal medicine in vivo tumor model of tumor inhibition s from a large number of natural medicine to find out, screening out of 48 kinds of anti-cancer invasion, metastasis, relapse traditional Chinese medicine

He participates in clinical validation and followed up for XZ - C immunoregulatory Chinese herbal medicine and completes the experimental research and clinical verification, data collection, collection and summary of this book.

A Brief Introduction to the Second Author

A brief introduction to the third author and the main translator and the main editor

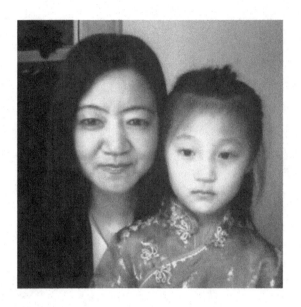

Bin Wu, MD, Ph.D., graduated from College of Yunyang of Tongji University of Medical Sciences for her MD degree; Studied her Master degree and her Ph. D degree in Sun Yat-Sen University of Medical Sciences. After she received her Ph.D., she worked as a Post-doctoral Follews in the Johns Hopkins Medical School and University of Maryland Medical School. She passed her USMLE tests and is going to do her residency training in America. She dedicated herself to oncology clinical and research. Her goal is to conquer cancer, which she believes this great contribution to our health. She has a daughter, named Lily Xu who drew all of the pictures in this book.

A Brief introduction to the illustrator and the advisor

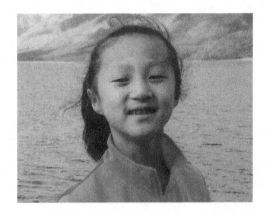

Lily Xu was born on November 17th 2006 and had an art presented in the Walter Art Museum in Baltimore at the age of 6; she got the fourth place trophy in the ES Double Digits or 24 and 24 games in the Baltimore County in Maryland; she got the first trophy in the BCPS STEM FAIR PHYSICS in Baltimore County; when she was in the sixth grade, she passed the advanced Math for 7th grade (which means the 8th grade math) test and moved the 8th grade math class; she loves the reading and writing and she finished many series of books. She got $6000 scholarship award for the Peabody music program in the Johns Hopkins University. In 2018 she was chosen into Baltimore county Middle school Honor Band. In 2018 the robotic team which she attended for years got designing-award from the Baltimore county so that this robotic team will come to Maryland State for the Robotic contest. On January 19th, 2019 she got the Robotic designing-award in Maryland . She edits all of my books for the publishing and drew all of the pictures in this book.

Acknowledgements

This book is for all of people who concern human being health. We are deeply grateful to all of people who like our new ways to improve our human being health.

My daughter **Lily Xu** gave me many smart and creative ideas while we were finishing this book. Lily Xu drew all of the pictures such as the Thymus etc. **The characteristics of she loves the challenge** and **her judgment always encourages me to continue working hard to move on**.

I would like to express our sincere gratitude to the following:

1. All of Authorhouse staffs
2. Dr. Xu Ze's family and Dr. Xu Jie's family, especially his son Zihao Xu, who is the medical student in China
3. Mrs. Bo Wu's family and Mrs. Tao Wu's famly: espeicaly their daughters Chongshu Luo and Xunyue Wang

Bin Wu, M.D., Ph.D
12-18-2018 in Baltimore, Maryland in USA

Foreword

Why did I take the title of the book as: "Walked out of a new road to overcome cancer", the title of the book is due to the guidance and inspiration from several experts, scholars, seniors, and teachers.

On July 2, 2001, Academician Wu Wei mentioned in his letter: "**The overall impression is: the mode from clinical to experimental and back from experimental to clinical is very good, the road of combining Chinese medicine with Western medicine is also very correct, I sincerely wish you keep moving forward and walk out of a new path to overcome cancer.**"

On February 22, 2006, Academician Tang Yu mentioned in his letter: "... **Chinese medicine and Chinese medication and biological therapy are the two most promising ways to resist metastasis, especially Chinese medication. I hope that you will walk out of the anti-metastasis road with Chinese characteristics.**"

On March 22, 2006, Academician Liu Yunyi mentioned in his letter: "...**I agree with your concept and thinking about cancer in your book... I hope that you can make a breakthrough contribution to traditional Chinese medicine again to make the benefits for the majority of patients and to make the traditional Chinese medicine be further developed, and to make my medical career reach a world status.**"

On January 9, 2006, Academician Wu Xianzhong mentioned in his letter: "...**the tumor is a difficult bone or the tumor is a hard bone, but it should continue to work on or it should continue to be continued. Fortunately, everyone is very objective, as long as it is effective, whether it is treating the tumor or the body, or reducing the reaction of the Chemotherapy or radiotherapy, the support will be given**. In the letter of April 10, 2012, "**We think that the road you have traveled is very special or very distinctive**. On the application formulation and the methods of taking or using and the drug combinations of the traditional Chinese medication, XZ-C drugs series have all innovated and developed and formed their own patents. **This road should continue to go or walk on.**"

Thanks for their guidance, guidance, and assistance in our research work, research thinking, research direction, research routes, research goals, and research methods. Thanks for their guidance, leading, and assistance in our research work, research thinking, research direction, research routes, research goals, and research methods. Our research work has been working in the direction of these guidance. I would like to express my gratitude to the academicians Wu Hao, Tang Wei, Wu Xianzhong and Liu Yunyi.

In the past 33 years (1985-present), cancer research has achieved a series of scientific and technological innovations and scientific research achievements in animal experimental research, clinical basic research and clinical verification. After more than 30 years of hard work, XZ-C immune regulation and control Anti-cancer treatment has been formed. In the past more than 30 years, a new road to conquer cancer has been taken out.

In the past 20 years, this series of experimental and clinical research work has received warm support and cordial guidance from Professor **Qiu Fazu**, who was the internationally renowned surgeon and the Master of the general surgery in China. In 1990, when the author submitted the "Eighth Five-Year Plan" key scientific and technological research project to the State Science and Technology Commission (the application of further exploring the anti-cancer and anti-metastasis experimental and clinical studies of cancer and anti-cancer Chinese herbal medicine for precancerous lesions of liver cancer and gastrointestinal cancer), Academician **Qiu Fazu** said in an expert opinion: **"It is a very important topic to study cancer metastasis and how to prevent metastasis. It is feasible to explore clinical prevention methods through experimental research and it is beneficial to people's work**." Under the meditate and guidance of the rigorous and scientific style of study of my teacher and Academican Qiu Fazu, we have completed the above projects, and I would like to thank you.

Scientific research must have nutritional feeding of the literature. In 1986, we just established an experimental surgical animal laboratory to make an animal model of cancer metastasis and conduct experimental research. We saw Professor Gao Jin's book "**Invasion and Metastasis of Cancer - Basic Research and Clinical Medicine**", and saw the monograph of Academician Tang Wei, "**Basic and Clinical Metastasis and Recurrence of Liver Cancer**". Theories in the two books make us suddenly see the light, or be clear. It also encourages and promotes our experimental work and clinical validation work from another aspect. Professor Tang Wei proposed in his monograph: **"The next important goal of primary liver cancer research - prevention and treatment of recurrence and metastasis**", and said: **"metastasis and recurrence have become a bottleneck to further improve the survival rate of liver cancer, and is one of the most important difficulties in combating cancer." These theoretical documents have given us the wisdom and courage to update our thinking and be brave in innovation, and have also strengthened the confidence and determination of our experimental team**. Here I would like to express my gratitude to Academician Tang Wei and Professor Gao Jin.

In the past 7 years, we have used more than 6,000 tumor-bearing animal models to explore one basic problem after another. The screening of 200 kinds of Chinese herbal medicines in the tumor-bearing animal model in vivo was carried out by several graduate students. Master Zhu Siping, Dr. Zou Shaomin, Master Li Zhengxun, Master of Liu Wei, etc., they carried out and completed a lot of hard and meticulous experimental work, take great pains, day and night, contributed to the development of experimental oncology medicine career for cancer prevention and anti-cancer. In hereI sincerely thank you all.

I. Over the past 30 years, it has walked out a new road of cancer treatment with immunomodulation of the combination of Chinese and Western medicine

First, the theoretical system of XZ-C immunomodulation and cancer treatment has been formed, and it has been undergoing the clinical application and observation verification.

(1)   cancer treatment concept
(2)   Cancer etiology and pathogenesis
(3)   Theoretical basis and experimental basis for cancer treatment
(4)   principles of cancer treatment
(5)   Cancer treatment mode
(6)   Principles of cancer metastasis treatment
(7)   New concept of cancer metastasis treatment
(8)   How to prevent cancer metastasis? Anti-cancer metastasis treatment "three steps"
(9)   Cancer treatment methods and drugs
(10) Research on new concepts and new methods of cancer metastasis treatment
(11) The formation of the theoretical system of XZ-C treatment

Contents

(1)   Concept of cancer treatment..9

    1. Traditional therapeutic concepts of cancer...............................9
    2. the new concept of cancer treatment 9

(2)   Cancer etiology and pathogenesis..13

    1. Thymus atrophy, immune dysfunction may be one of the causes and
       pathogenesis of cancer...13
    2. New findings in experimental research on the etiology, pathogenesis and
       pathophysiology of cancer...13
    3. Explore ways to curb tumor progression, progressive thymic atrophy, and
       immune reconstitution 13

(3)   Theoretical basis and experimental basis for cancer treatment 20

    1. Inspiration from animal experiments 20
    2. XZ-C immunomodulation therapy and the theoretical basis and experimental
       basis of " protection of Thymus and increase of immune function "........ 20
    3. It should protect, regulate and control, activate the body's anti-cancer immune
       system... 20
    4. Overview of research on anti-cancer Chinese medicines of similar biological
       modulators.. 20
    5. Biological response modifier-like action and efficacy of XZ-C
       immunoregulation of traditional Chinese medicines....................... 20

(4)   Principles of Cancer Treatment..28

    1. Principles of cancer treatment – it should change the concept and establish a
       comprehensive treatment concept...28
    2. the traditional therapy target is simple, only kill cancer cells..............28
    3. traditional therapy ignores the host's own resistance to cancer...........28
    4. Initiative to establish a comprehensive treatment perspective for both tumors
       and hosts 28

5. how to establish a comprehensive treatment concept of cancer 28
6. immune regulation is also the focus of comprehensive treatment of cancer 28

(5) Cancer treatment mode..37

1. Why is there a new model for organic comprehensive treatment? 37
2. How to formulate a new multi-disciplinary organic comprehensive treatment model 37
3. Initiatives for specific programs for multidisciplinary treatment of cancer.................37

(6) Principles of cancer metastasis treatment.. 44

1. cancer research or conquering cancer, the key is anti-metastasis 44
2. the basic principle of cancer treatment is anti-metastasis...................................... 44
3. The main feature of the new concept of cancer treatment, namely control transfer.... 44
4. One of the goals of 21st century cancer treatment should be anti-metastasis.............. 44
5. "If it didn't research or study cancer metastasis, improving the efficacy would
   be an empty talk."... 44

(7) New concept of cancer metastasis treatment 48

1. The main manifestations of cancer in the human body or the main existing
   form of cancer in the human body...48
2. Traditional cancer therapies believe that there are two forms 48
3. The new concept of cancer treatment is considered to have three forms.......................48
4. The third form of research and understanding process of cancer in human body 48
5. The research and understanding of the third form of cancer in the human body........48
6. the goal of cancer treatment should be directed to the above three forms of existence...48
7. <u>To target or aim cancer cells on the way will bring a new dawn for conquering
   cancer or the fight against cancer</u>...48

(8) How to stop or prevent cancer metastasis? "three steps" of anti-cancer metastasis
     treatment 54

1. The steps of cancer metastasis should be understood so that it makes the cancer
   treatment goals more specific...54
2. Try to break each metastasis step one by one..54
3. Three major countermeasures for anti-cancer metastasis treatment ("Three Steps")....54

(9) Cancer treatment methods and drugs 59

1. Experimental research work:...60
   In vivo anti-tumor screening test...60
2. Clinical observation, verification 61
   Based on the success of animal experiments, clinical application verification..............61

3. *The series of XZ-C immune regulation and control anti-cancer Chinese medicine.....63*

(10) *Research on new concepts and new methods of cancer metastasis treatment 77*

(11) *The formation of the theoretical system of XZ-C immune regulation and treatment of cancer 87*

Walked out of the new road of cancer treatment with the immune regulation and control of the combination of Chinese and Western medicine

——XZ-C immunomodulation anticancer treatment has been formed

For more than 60 years, the new road to conquer cancer has been taken out.

First, the theoretical system of XZ-C immunomodulation cancer treatment has been formed, and it has been undergoing clinical application and observation verification.

(1) cancer treatment concept (introduction)

1. The traditional concept holds that cancer is the continuous division and proliferation of cancer cells, and its therapeutic goal must be to kill cancer cells. **Therefore, the traditional therapeutic concept of cancer is based on the killing of cancer cells.** In order to achieve cure, the last cancer cell must be killed, so people have used extended surgery, intensive chemotherapy and radical radiotherapy, but the results are not satisfactory.
2. a new model of cancer treatment believes that: **cure should be through regulation and control rather than single kill**, the final step in curing cancer is to mobilize the reproduction of host control, rather than destroy the last cancer cells.

1

Concept of cancer treatment (introduction)

1.   Traditional therapeutic concepts of cancer
2.   the new concept of cancer treatment

1.   Traditional therapeutic concepts of cancer

The traditional therapeutic concept holds that cancer is the continuous division and proliferation of cancer cells, and its therapeutic goal must be to kill cancer cells. Therefore, the goal of the traditional three major treatments is based on the killing of cancer cells.

The basic principle of traditional cancer treatment is that the last cancer cell must be killed or eliminated. Therefore, people have used extended surgery, intensive chemotherapy and radical radiotherapy. But the results are not ideal. In the early 1960s, the scope of oncology surgery expanded and a series of ultra-radical procedures were developed. After many years of practice, the expansion of surgical resection, such as breast cancer, lung cancer, liver cancer, and pancreatic cancer, did not change the patient's cancer-free survival and overall survival. In the 1980s, intensive chemotherapy and radical radiotherapy did not improve the quality of life or prolong survival. On the contrary, due to the severe inhibition of bone marrow hematopoietic function and immune function, some life-threatening complications were increased. This suggests that it may be necessary to establish a new model, try to explore from other angles, update ideas, and find new ways.

In short, the traditional concept that cancer is based on cell mad division and proliferation, cancer cells are the culprit. Therefore, in traditional cancer therapy, the target of treatment is set as cancer cells, and the goal is to kill cancer cells.

2.   **The new concept of cancer treatment**

Healing should be through regulation and control rather than killed.

The dominant idea of the new model of cancer is that the regulation and signaling between cells in cancer patients is disrupted rather than lost; it is believed that carcinogenesis is a continuum with reversal potential.

The new model for cancer is based on information transfer and regulatory control. It acknowledges that malignant transformation is a process of gradual progress, but also believes that they have the potential to reverse. **The new model of cancer believes that healing should be regulated and controlled rather than killed.**

Note: "Monograph" - "New Concepts and New Methods for Cancer Treatment" (the third monograph of Professor Xu Ze (XU ZE)"

The experience of clinical practice and experimental research suggests that we: there is some response relationship between the tumor and the host. If the tumor is seen as the result of a regulatory imbalance, rather than the autonomic behavior of the tumor, some clinical phenomena are easier to understand. **We know that clinically, tumor cells can respond highly to the host's environment. Long-term application of immunosuppressive drugs can induce tumors, and when the immunosuppressive drugs are stopped, the tumors can be completely relieved**. Although the factors that induce tumors have not been confirmed, <u>**the host response determines the final outcome. Renal tumors with lung metastasis can be completely relieved after stopping anti-rejection therapy. Pregnancy also seems to change the relationship between the tumor and the host.**</u> Looking at the killing of tumors, people have developed a variety of treatment methods for half a century, and developed many anti-cancer drugs, but still failed to prevent tumor invasion and metastasis. From the current data, cytotoxic drug-assisted chemotherapy after surgery also failed to prevent cancer recurrence and metastasis. Because it mostly has a serious inhibitory effect on immunity, it can even inhibit the non-immune part of the host reaction. When we perform intensive chemotherapy, it is likely to cause artificial or iatrogenic immune failure.

Now, from the perspective of molecular biology, cancer is a change in the structure of cellular DNA, which is a disorder of cell differentiation caused by changes in genetic information. The introduction of normal nucleic acid into tumor cells by genetic engineering can induce differentiation of tumor cells into normal cells. The Shanghai Cancer Institute has extracted ribonucleic acid from normal liver cells and incubated with hepatocytes. Through the regulation of normal liver ribonucleic acid, the abnormality of gene activity of liver cancer cells can be corrected, leading to reversal of normal cells. Science is looking for living active substances related to genetic information, such as normal information RNA (mRNA) can induce cancer cells to reverse to normal cells.

The use of cytotoxic drugs to treat cancer is based on the fact that the last cancer cell must be killed until the tumor is clinically and laboratoryly proven to be completely eliminated. But based on our 20 years of experience, there are still many contradictions in this view. There are some clinical examples that use a killing method to shrink or subside a tumor, but it is not necessarily a direct cure. As the dose of cytotoxic drugs continues to increase, most patients' cancer cells begin to subside, but the patient's survival rate does not improve, and soon will relapse and the tumor will increase.

It seems that patients who have been cured are not using killing cells. **For example, platinum** drugs treat tumors and appear to be involved in inducing cell differentiation. The effects of interferon and interleukin on sensitive cells also play a role through regulatory mechanisms. As adjunctive therapy for colorectal cancer, the effect of levamisole is considered to be a change from the host response.

In the past, we tried our best to treat cancer cells, but it did not achieve great success. Extended radical, intensive chemotherapy and radical radiotherapy have been used. However, the results are not ideal and fail to improve the quality of life of cancer patients and prolong the survival of cancer patients.

In the past 60 years, Chinese medicine has achieved great results in the treatment of cancer. A large amount of data reported in various places indicates that cancer cells can coexist with the host, and the host has a long survival period. In the past 16 years, more than 12,000 patients with advanced cancer in the Shuguang Cancer Research Institute and Wuchang Shuguang Oncology Clinic have been relapsed and metastatic patients, such as anastomotic recurrence cancer, gastric cancer, and can not be resected and can not be treated with radiotherapy or chemotherapy. Long-term treatment of XZ-C immunomodulation of traditional Chinese medicine for 3-5 years, the disease can be controlled, stable tumor-bearing survival (coexistence with cancer), life is completely self-care, quality of life is good, and survival is significantly prolonged.

We believe that the foreigners who invade the body should undoubtedly carry out ruthless killing. Then, the treatment of cancer cells is different, because they are only the mutated tissues in the normal body of the host itself. Therefore, cancer should be controlled by adjusting the body. **It is not necessary or impossible to kill all cancer cells.**

Because of the new understanding of the concept of cancer, the concept of cancer therapy should also update ideas, update understanding, and then innovate treatment theory and technology.

In view of the author's half-century experience, we should seek breakthroughs in clinical research from the urgent problems of current cancer research and the weakness of modern medicine, and seek breakthroughs in prevention and treatment from invasion, recurrence and metastasis, from chemical synthetic drugs and natural medicines and perform targeted treatment at the molecular level, gene level, and comprehensive treatment level to deepen the new understanding of the concept of cancer.

(2) <u>Cancer etiology and pathogenesis (introduction)</u>

In order to explore the etiology, pathogenesis and pathophysiology of cancer, we conducted a series of animal experiments, analyzing and thinking from the experimental results, so that we can obtain new discoveries, new thinking, new enlightenment: thymus atrophy, immune dysfunction It is one of the causes and pathogenesis of cancer. Therefore, Professor XU ZE proposed one of the causes and pathogenesis of cancer at international conferences, which may be thymus atrophy, impaired central immune function, immune function, immune surveillance. Reduced ability and immune escape. *After the investigation, this is the first time in the world. (See Chapter 2 of this book)*

2

Cancer etiology and pathogenesis (introduction)

1. Thymus atrophy, immune dysfunction may be one of the causes and pathogenesis of cancer
2. *New findings in experimental research on the etiology, pathogenesis and pathophysiology of cancer*
3. *Explore ways to curb tumor progression, progressive thymic atrophy, and immune reconstitution*

1. New findings in experimental research on the etiology, pathogenesis and pathophysiology of cancer

In the past 16 years, the author has carried out a series of experimental studies on exploring the possible etiology, pathogenesis and pathophysiology of cancer, exploring the mechanisms of cancer invasion, recurrence and metastasis, and looking for effective measures for regulation.

Experimental surgery is extremely important in the development of medical science. It is a key to opening the medical exclusion zone. Many disease prevention methods are applied to the clinic after many animal experiments have achieved stability results. Therefore, the author established an experimental surgical laboratory to conduct experimental tumor research, implement cancer cell transplantation, establish a tumor animal model, and carried out the following series of experimental tumor research: 1 to explore the experimental study of cancer etiology, pathogenesis, pathophysiology; 2 to explore cancer Recurrence, metastasis mechanism and regularity; 3 to explore the relationship between tumor and immune and immune organs, and immune organs and tumors; 4 to explore ways to curb tumor progression, progressive atrophy of immune organs and immune reconstitution; 5 to find out the effective measures for the regulation and control of cancer invasion, recurrence and metastasis.

From the experimental tumor research, in order to explore the etiology, pathogenesis, invasion and metastasis mechanism of cancer, and to find effective measures for regulation, intervention,

Authors: Xu Ze (China) ; Xu Jie(China) ; Bin Wu(America)

invasion, recurrence and metastasis, the author and colleagues conducted a full four-year experimental tumor research work.

(1) Experiment 1: Excision of mouse thymus (Thymus, TH) to produce a tumor-bearing animal model, injection of immunosuppressive drugs contribute to the establishment of a cancer-bearing animal model. **The conclusion of the study proves that the occurrence and development of cancer have a significant correlation with the thymus and its function of the host immune organs**.

(2) Experiment 2: Whether it is immune first and then easy to get cancer, or cancer first and then low immunity, the experimental results confirmed: first, the immune system is low and then easy to have cancer, the development, if no immune function decline, it is not easy to vaccinate success. The results suggest that improving and maintaining good immune function and protecting the central thymus gland is one of the important measures to prevent cancer.

(3) Experiment 3: In the study of the relationship between metastasis and immunity of cancer, an animal model of liver metastasis was established and divided into two groups, A and B groups. Group A used immunosuppressive drugs, and group B did not. Results The number of intrahepatic metastases in group A was significantly higher than that in group B. The experimental results suggest that metastasis is related to immunity, and low immune function or application of immunosuppressive drugs may promote tumor metastasis.

(4) Experiment 4: When investigating the effect of tumor on the immune organs of the body, it was found that the thymus was progressively atrophied as the cancer progressed, and the host thymus was acute progressive atrophy after the cancer cells were swollen, and cell proliferation was blocked. The volume is significantly reduced. The experimental results suggest that the tumor may inhibit the thymus and cause the immune organs to shrink.

(5) Experiment 5: It was found in the experiment that some of the experimental mice did not have a successful vaccination or the tumor grew very small, and the thymus did not significantly shrink. To understand the relationship between tumor and thymus atrophy, a group of experimental mice transplanted solid tumors were resected when they reached the size of the thumb. After 1 month of dissection, it was found that the thymus did not undergo progressive atrophy. Therefore, we speculate that a solid tumor may produce a factor that is not yet known to inhibit the thymus, which needs further study.

(6) Experiment 6: The above experimental results all prove that the progression of the tumor can cause progressive atrophy of the thymus, then can some methods be used to prevent the host thymus from shrinking? Through animal experiments, we began to find ways or drugs to prevent thymocyte atrophy in tumor-bearing mice. The immune organ cells were transplanted to restore the function of the immune organs, and the methods of suppressing tumor progression, thymus atrophy of immune organs, and immune reconstruction were adopted. Rats were transplanted with fetal liver, fetal spleen and fetal thymus cells, and experimental studies on the immune function of adoptive immune reconstitution. The results showed that: S, T, L three groups of cells combined

transplantation, the recent complete tumor regression rate was 40%, the long-term tumor complete regression rate was 46.67%, the tumor completely disappeared long-term survival.

(7) Experiment 7: In the experiment to investigate the effect of tumor on the spleen of the immune organs of the body, it was found that the spleen had an inhibitory effect on tumor growth in the early stage of the tumor, and in the late stage of the tumor, the spleen also showed progressive atrophy. The results suggest that the effect of spleen on tumor growth is bidirectional, with some inhibition in the early stage and no inhibition in the late stage. Spleen cell transplantation can enhance the inhibition of tumors.

(8) Experiment 8: The results of follow-up suggest that controlled metastasis is the key to cancer treatment. Currently, there are many steps and links in cancer cell transfer. In order to try to block one of the links to prevent its metastasis, it is considered that tumor neovascularization is one of the links in which metastatic cancer cells can grow into a cancer nodule. In the year, the author carried out microcirculation research, observed microvascular formation and flow velocity of transplanted tumor nodules in mice with microcirculation microscopy, and then searched for anti-tumor blood vessels from natural drugs and then from natural drugs. The formed drug was observed through the Olympus microcirculation micro-photography system to observe the neovascularization process and count the flow rate of the micro-arteries and venules, and the ethyl acetate extract (TG) was screened. The results showed that there was no neovascularization on the first day of inoculation, and on the second day, microscopic neovascularization was observed. TG can reduce the density of new microvessels entering and leaving the tumor.

(9) Experiment 9: It was found from a large number of tumor-bearing animal models in the laboratory that the solid tumors inoculated subcutaneously in the experimental mice were larger, and the central tissues of the cancer cells were different from the surrounding cancer cells, and the nodule centers were more For sterile necrosis or liquefaction, the surrounding area is still active cancer cells. Therefore, in the clinical treatment work, the treatment of sterile necrosis can be taken.

2. To explore ways to curb the progression of cancer, progressive atrophy of the thymus, and reconstruction of immunity.

From the above experimental studies, one of the causes of cancer and the pathogenesis may be thymus atrophy, thymocyte proliferation is blocked, thymus function is impaired, and immune function is low, leading to immune escape of malignant cells.

Since the thymus develops progressive atrophy as the tumor progresses, how do you intervene to prevent it from shrinking? Animal experimental studies were conducted to find ways or drugs to prevent thymic atrophy in tumor-bearing mice, and finally transplanted with immune organ cells to restore the function of the immune organs, and achieved exciting results.

Authors: Xu Ze (China) ; Xu Jie(China) ; Bin Wu(America)

At that time, the author had considered the above-mentioned experimental methods for clinical trials, trying to use the water-sacs to induce the thymus homogenate to try the allogeneic thymocyte transplantation, but medical ethics is not allowed, so it was not implemented.

In 1986, at a satellite conference of the International Microcirculation Conference, the author was inspired from the discussion for finding microcirculatory drugs from natural medicines, then turn or shift from biological cell transplantation, adoptive immunization to rebuild immune, and then look for activation from natural medicines of Chinese herbal medicine. Cytokines enhance immune surveillance, thereby inhibiting tumors and preventing thymic atrophy. All drugs must pass animal experiments and clinical verification, so in the research of animal models of cancer-bearing animals, after more than 3 years, more than 200 kinds of odor-suppressing screening experiments were carried out from natural Chinese herbal medicines. Finally, the anti-cancer immune regulation Chinese herbal medicine which has a good tumor suppressing effect is screened out. After clinical screening and clinical verification, it is further screened from Chinese medicine immunopharmacology and concentrated into XZ-C1-10 anti-cancer immune regulation Chinese medicine, which can promote thymic hyperplasia, prevent thymus atrophy, enhance immune function and protect bone marrow and promote T lymphocyte function and cytokines, and have a high tumor inhibition rate, only inhibit cancer cells without affecting normal cells, and can be taken orally for a long time. Because cancer is a chronic disease, the division, proliferation, and cloning of cancer cells are long-term, continuous, and progressive. Therefore, it is recommended to use long-term, non-toxic, orally administrable sustained-release drugs. Chinese herbal medicine for treating cancer is to treat the cause and mechanism of the disease from the overall point of view of human beings. It not only kills cancer cells, but also enhances the body's autoimmune function, thereby enhancing the body's anti-cancer ability, so it can make some refractory, The widespread transfer of cancer is controlled, prolonging the lives of cancer patients, alleviating the suffering of patients, and opening up a path worthy of further exploration for cancer treatment.

The results of a series of animal experiments on the etiology, pathogenesis and pathophysiology of cancer suggest that thymectomy leads to immunodeficiency, and then the immune surveillance declines, eventually developing into immune escape, which may be one of the key factors of cancer etiology and pathogenesis. It is a new development of 21st century oncology theory, which provides direction and basis for cancer therapeutics in the 21st century, and provides theoretical basis and experimental basis for cancer immune regulation and targeted therapy. This innovation has not been mentioned in textbooks and literature at home and abroad.

Once the above theory and doctrine have been demonstrated and recognized, it will lead to a series of changes and updates in cancer therapeutics, such as changes and updates in the understanding of the concept of cancer treatment, changes and updates in the understanding of cancer treatment goals or targets, and diagnosis of cancer. Changes and updates in methodological and therapeutic criteria, changes and updates in cancer treatment methods and treatment models; changes and updates in the research and development of anticancer and anti-metastatic drugs.

The Research of New Concept and Way of Treatment of Carcinoma

In 1985, the author surveyed more than 3000 cases of thoracic and abdominal surgeries made by him and found that relapse and metastasis are the key factors that affect postoperative curative effects.

↓

It is necessary to do basic clinical research to prevent relapse and metastasis

↓

The author built a laboratory foe animal experiments

↓

Made cancer-bearing animal model

↓

New findings from the experimental research

↓

| Finding 1: Ablating thymus can make cancer-bearing animal model | Finding 2: Immunosuppressant can weaken immunity to make the model | Finding 3: Thymus atrophy with the evolvement of cancer | Finding 4: Metastasis is related to immunity; weak immunity may accelerate metastasis | Finding 5: For the inoculated mice, their thymuses shrink progressively; those without inoculation, there is no thymus atrophy. Ablate he thymus when it grows to the size like finger tip | Finding 6: Tumors can inhibit thymus and lead to atrophy of immune organs. So it can be predicted that solid tumors can produce some kind of factor to inhibit TH, called factor of inhibiting thymus by cancer cells. |

↓

From the above findings, it can be known that the evolution of tumors can make immune organs progressive atrophy and decrease immunity progressively.

↓

How to prevent TH atrophy?
How to promote immune surveillance?
The following research has been done in the laboratory

↓

17

Authors: Xu Ze (China) ; Xu Jie(China) ; Bin Wu(America)

How to avoid thymus atrophy? How to avoid exhaustion of immunity?	How to prevent thymus atrophy? How to protect immune organs? How to strengthen immunity and avoid exhaustion of immunity

Immunologic reconstitution by adoptive immunity through transplantation of fetal liver, thymus and spleen cell	Look for the medicament that can prevent thymus atrophy and strengthen immunity.

The experimental results indicate that in the group of combined transplantation of S, T, L cells, the complete regression rate in near future is 40% and that of forward future is 46.67%. Those with regression can survive for a long time with good curative effects.	Screen 200 kinds of traditional Chinese medicines by experiments to find out the medicine that can protect thymus and strengthen immunity, promote hematopiesis and resist relapse and metastasis.

Experimental articles can not be published	The experiments for screening in the laboratory for three years: 1) screening experiment by the rate of inhibiting tumors in vitro; 2) screening experiment by the rate of inhibiting tumors in vivo of cancer-bearing animal model

Screen and look for natural medicament from traditional Chinese herbs through animal experiment.	From a series of experimental research on tumors with cancer-bearing animals over 7 years, there is a deeply-felt that it is necessary to persist in research on resisting cancerometastasis with Chinese characteristics, namely the combination of experimental research and clinical verification. It is essential to do experimental research on tumors, or it is difficult to improve clinical curative effects.

(3) Theoretical basis and experimental basis for cancer treatment

As a result of laboratory experiments, it was found that the thymus of the cancer-bearing mice showed progressive atrophy, and the function of the central immune organ was impaired, the immune function was decreased, and the immune surveillance was low. **Therefore, the treatment principle must be to prevent progressive atrophy of the thymus and promote thymic hyperplasia. It protects the bone marrow hematopoietic function, improves immune surveillance, and controls the immune escape of malignant cells.**

Based on the above findings on the experimental results of cancer etiology and pathogenesis, it is a new theory and method for XZ-C immunomodulation therapy. After 34 years of clinical trials of more than 12,000 patients with advanced cancer in 60 years of oncology clinic, the author confirmed that the treatment principle of protection of thymus and increase of immune function is reasonable and satisfactory.

XZ-C (XU ZE – China) immunomodulatory therapy was first proposed by Professor Xu Ze in his book "New Concepts and New Methods of Cancer Metastasis Treatment" in 2006. **He believes that under normal circumstances, there is a dynamic balance between cancer and body defense; the occurrence of cancer is the imbalance of dynamic balance. If the state of the disorder has been adjusted to a normal level, the growth of the cancer can be controlled and allowed to subside.**

It is well known that the occurrence, development and prognosis of cancer are determined by the comparison of two factors, namely, the biological characteristics of cancer cells and the host body's own ability to control cancer cells. **If the two are balanced, the cancer can be controlled, and if the two are out of balance, the cancer develops.**

Under normal circumstances, the host's body itself **has certain restrictive ability to cancer cells**, but in the case of cancer, these restrictive defense capabilities are inhibited and damaged to varying degrees, resulting in cancer cells losing immune surveillance and cellular immune escape. The cancer cells are further developed and metastasized.

(See Chapter 3 of the book, P17)

3

Theoretical basis and experimental basis for cancer treatment (introduction)

Theoretical basis and experimental basis of XZ-C immunomodulatory therapy of protection of Thymus and enhancement of immune function

1. Inspiration from animal experiments
2. XZ-C immunomodulation therapy and the theoretical basis and experimental basis of " protection of Thymus and increase of immune function "
3. It should protect, regulate and control, activate the body's anti-cancer immune system
4. Overview of research on anti-cancer Chinese medicines of similar biological modulators
5. Biological response modifier-like action and efficacy of XZ-C immunoregulation of traditional Chinese medicines

1. Inspiration from animal experiments

The author's laboratory found that the thymus of the cancer-bearing mice showed progressive atrophy and the central immune organs were damaged, so the treatment should be protected by "protecting the thymus and increasing immune function" to protect the thymus and boost immunity.

Based on the results of experimental research on the etiology and pathogenesis of cancer, Professor Xu Ze first proposed a new theory and method for XZ-C immunomodulation targeted therapy. **As a result of the experimental study, it was found that the cancer-bearing mice had progressive atrophy of the thymus, and the central immune organ function was impaired, the immune function was decreased, and the immune surveillance was low. Therefore, the treatment principle should be to prevent progressive atrophy of the thymus and promote thymic hyperplasia, protect bone marrow hematopoietic function, improve immune surveillance, and control immune escape of malignant cells.**

It is well known that the immune organs have central immune organs and peripheral immune organs. The former is the thymus and bone marrow, and the latter is the spleen and lymph nodes. It has been confirmed that when cancer occurs, **a factor that inhibits the immune organs [we temporarily call it a cancer suppressing or inhibiting Thymus (inhibiting immune function) factor]** inhibits the thymus, causes the thymus to gradually shrink, and the central immune function is inhibited, and thus the immune function. Decline, the immune surveillance is weakened or missing, and the tumor will inevitably develop further.

After 34 years of clinical trials of more than 12,000 patients with advanced cancer in the oncology clinic, the author has confirmed that the treatment principle of breast enhancement is correct and reasonable, and the curative effect is satisfactory.

Note: "Monograph" - "New Concepts and New Methods of Cancer Therapy" (the third monograph of Professor Xu Ze"

XZ-C (XU ZE-China) immunomodulatory therapy was first proposed by Professor Xu Ze in China in 2006 in his book "New Concepts and New Methods for Cancer Metastasis Treatment". He believes that under normal circumstances, there is a dynamic balance between cancer and body defense. The occurrence and development of cancer is caused by the imbalance of dynamic balance. If the condition that has been dysregulated is adjusted to a normal level, the growth of the cancer can be controlled and allowed to subside.

It is well known that the occurrence and development of cancer and its prognosis are determined by the comparison of two factors, namely, the biological characteristics of cancer cells and the host body's own ability to control cancer cells. If the balance between the two is cancer, the cancer can be controlled. Unbalance is the development of cancer.

Under normal circumstances, the host's body itself has certain restrictions on cancer cells, but in the case of cancer, these restrictive defenses are inhibited and damaged to varying degrees, resulting in cancer cells losing immune surveillance and cancer cells. Immune escape, allowing cancer cells to further develop and metastasize.

2. **It should protect, regulate, activate the body's anti-cancer immune system**

When discussing the principles of cancer treatment, we should study what anti-cancer immune cell series are in the human body, what anti-cancer cell factor series are, what anti-cancer gene series are, and which humoral immunity series are.

(1) What anti-cancer immune cells in the human body may be activated and enhanced to prevent cancer cell metastasis:

(A) Cytotoxic lymphocytes (CTL): play a major role in anti-tumor immunity. Human CTL cells are CD3 and CD8. CTL cells are high in peripheral blood and spleen, in thoracic duct, thymus, and bone marrow. There is a certain amount. Under certain conditions, IL-2, IL-4, IFN and other cytokines can also be produced, and other anti-cancer immune cells, killing macrophages, natural killer cells and killer B cells can be activated to exert anti-tumor effects.

(B) Natural killer cells (NK cells): NK cells are a group of broad-spectrum anti-cancer cells whose killing activity is independent of antibodies and does not depend on the thymus. Its main function is to monitor and eliminate cancerous cells in the human body. Clinical observations have found that the incidence of malignant tumors is significantly increased in people with NK activity deficiency, and NK cells are an important part of the early anti-cancer immune surveillance function of the body.

(C) LAK cells: LAK cells are the most important anti-cancer cells in modern biological therapy. Human peripheral monocytes (PBMNC) can significantly kill a variety of tumor cells in vitro induced by IL-2 in vitro. LAK cells have a broader spectrum of tumorigenicity than NK cells and can also kill tumor cells that NK cells cannot kill.

(D) Macrophages (MΦ): It plays an important role in the body's anti-tumor immunity.

(2) What anti-cancer cell factors in the human body can be activated and enhanced to prevent cancer metastasis

(A) Interferon (IFN): Interferon is capable of resisting cell differentiation and has an immunoregulatory function. It has anti-proliferative effects on certain tumor cells, and its anti-cancer effect may be related to immune regulation. It enhances the activity of NK cells and MΦ cells.

(B) Interleukin-2 (IL-2): It is a T cell growth factor with strong immunoregulatory function, which promotes the activation of T cells, NK cells and monocytes, and also promotes IFN-a and TNF. Release.

(C) Tumor necrosis factor (TNF): its effect on cells is cytotoxic and can affect the microvessels of the tumor, eventually leading to necrosis of the central part of the tumor.

(3) Others

In recent years, due to the rapid development of molecular biology, molecular immunology, molecular immunopharmacology, and genetic engineering, the basic and clinical research of the molecular level of "anti-cancer institutions" has been continuously expanded and deepened.

At present, research on anti-cancer molecular biological immunotherapy mainly focuses on four subsystems of anti-cancer institutions, namely anti-cancer therapy, anti-cancer factor therapy, anti-cancer gene therapy and anti-cancer antibody therapy.

The basic feature of these molecular biology and molecular immunotherapy is that all preparations of molecular biological immunotherapy are the organism's own substances. The fundamental difference between it and the radiotherapy and chemotherapy is that it is normal to the body's normal tissue cells, especially to the immune system. The system's cells and functions, the structure and function of the bone marrow hematopoietic system, not only have no progressive damage, but also have immune response regulation and enhancement. It is well known that radiotherapy and chemotherapy are non-selective "invasive therapies". Killing cancer cells also kills normal cells, which can damage the normal tissue cells of the body, causing serious damage to the bone marrow hematopoietic system and immune structure and function, leading to serious consequences.

Biological therapy is a therapy that stabilizes and balances the life mechanism through regulation of biological responses. American scholar Oldham proposed the theory of biological regulation in 1984, and then proposed the concept of tumor biological therapy.

3. Overview of research on immunomodulation anti-cancer Chinese medicines of similar biological modulators

XZ-C immunomodulation anti-cancer Chinese medicine has been confirmed by animal experiments and clinical practice to have bio-regulatory-like effects and curative effects, and is a drug selected from natural medicine resources.

The experimental screening work was mainly carried out by the in vivo anti-tumor experiment of the tumor-bearing animal model. One experimental group of traditional Chinese medicine was observed. The animal model was observed for 3 months, and 48 effective anti-cancer Chinese herbal medicines were selected for each 2 or 3 flavors. In vivo anti-tumor experiments of tumor-bearing animals were carried out. It was found that the anti-tumor experiment of single-flavor Chinese medicine was not as good as the anti-tumor effect of the compound anti-tumor experiment of multi-flavored traditional Chinese medicine, and the single-flavor Chinese medicine only inhibited the proliferation of tumors. The compound combination of multi-flavored traditional Chinese medicine not only inhibits the tumor growth of tumor-bearing animals, but also has a good regulation effect on immune regulation, enhancement of physical strength, enhancement of immune function, promotion of tumor cell cytokine production and protection of normal cells.

On the basis of the in vitro experimental screening of the traditional Chinese medicine in the early stage of 4 years and the screening of the tumor-inhibiting model in the tumor-bearing animal model, the experimental combination was optimized, and then the experiment was reconstituted to XZ-C1-10 immunoregulation, anti-cancer, anti-metastasis, Anti-relapse combination, and finally clinical validation. Since 1992, the author has organized a collaborative group to carry out clinical verification. After 16 years of clinical trials and observations of more than 12,000 patients with various cancers in the Twilight Oncology Clinic, the patients have stable, improved symptoms, improved symptoms, improved quality of life, and survival. The period is significantly extended. Many patients who have metastasized stabilized the lesion after taking the drug. The cancer cells did not spread and metastasize further. Some patients could not undergo radiotherapy or chemotherapy for reasons such as decreased white blood cell count after surgery, and the metastasis was controlled after taking the drug, and no metastasis was observed.

4. **Biological response modifier-like action and efficacy of XZ-C immunoregulation of traditional Chinese medicines**

The regulation of biological responses was first described by Oldham in 1982. The implication is the ability to regulate the body's response or response to an external "attack" through a biological response modifier (BRM).

The cells and humoral factors of the body's immune system **are in a delicate regulation and control**. In the case of loss of balance, the body's response or response ability will be significantly affected. The use of biological response modifiers is to restore the balance of the body state to normal balance, in order to achieve the purpose of disease prevention.

BRM opens up new areas of cancer biotherapy. At present, BRM is widely regarded as the fourth mode of cancer treatment by the medical community.

The biological response modifier has the function of regulating and controlling the body's immune function and restoring the suppressed immune system of the body. Its mechanism of action is multifaceted, but no matter what mechanism, it plays its regulatory role by activating the body's immune system.

Biological response modifiers, mostly microbial and plant sources, formerly known as immunopotentiators, immune cordial, immunostimulants or immunomodulators, are now collectively designated as biological response modifiers or modifiers.

In the laboratory, the XZ-C immunomodulatory anti-cancer anti-metastasis Chinese medicine which has a good tumor inhibition rate in the laboratory has improved immunity, protects the central immune organ thymus, enhances cellular immunity, and protects thymus tissue function and improves immunity, protects bone marrow blood production, increases red blood cell and white blood cell count, activates immune cytokines, and improves immune surveillance in the blood. The main pharmacological action of XZ-C immunomodulation anticancer Chinese medicine is the protection of Thymus and the enhancement of immune function. 48 kinds of traditional Chinese medicines that have been screened out in 4 years of animal experiments and have a high tumor inhibition rate. After detection by immunological and cytokine levels, 26 of them were able to enhance phagocytosis; or enhance cellular immunity; or enhance humoral immunity; or increase the weight of the thymus; or promote bone marrow cell proliferation; or enhance T cell function; or enhance LAK cell activity;

or inhibit platelet coagulation and antithrombotic; or antiviral, anti-metastatic; or remove free radicals and other effects. **To summarize the anti-cancer mechanism of XZ-C immunomodulation anti-cancer Chinese medicine is:**

(1) Activate the immune cell system of the body, promote the enhancement of the effect of the host defense mechanism, and restore the ability to respond to cancer.

(2) Activate the immune cytokine system of the body's anti-cancer mechanism, enhance the host's immune defense mechanism, and improve the immune surveillance of the immune system of the body's blood circulation system.

(3) Protect the thymus, enhance immunity, protect the marrow from blood, protect the bone marrow physiological mechanism, stimulate the bone marrow hematopoietic

function, promote the recovery of bone marrow function, and improve the white blood cell and red blood cell count.

(4)   to alleviate the adverse reactions of radiotherapy and chemotherapy, and enhance the tolerance of the host.

(5)   The progression of cancer is caused by the imbalance between the biological characteristics of cancer cells and the body's ability to inhibit cancer. The immune regulation of XZ-C is to improve immunity and restore balance.

(6)   It can directly regulate the growth and differentiation of tumor cells, and regulate the growth and differentiation.

(7)   The thymus can be enlarged and gained, so that the thymus does not undergo progressive atrophy.

(8)   Stimulate the host's anti-tumor immune response, enhance the body's anti-tumor ability, enhance the sensitivity of cancer cells to the body's anti-cancer mechanism, and help to kill cancer cells on the way to metastasis.

XZ-C immunomodulation of traditional Chinese medicine treatment of tumors can enable the host to produce a strong immune response to cancer cells, thereby achieving the purpose of treating cancer. XZ-C immunomodulation anticancer Chinese medicine can cause the following immunological reactions in the host: 1 enhance the regulation or restore the host's immune response to the tumor; 2 stimulate the body's inherent immune function, activate the host's immune defense system; 3 restore immune function.

As mentioned above, the mechanism of action of XZ-C immunomodulation anticancer Chinese medicine is basically similar to that of BRM, and the clinical use also has the same therapeutic effect as BRM.

(4) principles of cancer treatment (introduction)

Cancer treatment should change the concept and establish a comprehensive treatment concept. The author believes that cancer treatment should overcome the current one-sided treatment concept aimed at killing cancer cells, change concepts, and establish a comprehensive treatment concept. Traditional therapy targets are simple, killing only cancer cells, but neglecting the host's own resistance to cancer cells. Therefore, we advocate the establishment of a comprehensive treatment perspective for both tumors and hosts. It is necessary to establish a new treatment mode to achieve better therapeutic results.

After deep thought, the author put forward the concept of "balance theory" that affects the occurrence and development of cancer.

If the target of treatment only kills cancer cells, but only for one aspect, it is impossible to overcome cancer if it is a one-sided treatment concept. The goal of treatment should be to target both the host and the cancer cells, both to kill cancer cells and protect the host, enhance immunity, protect the chest from lifting, protect the marrow from blood, and enhance the host's ability to fight cancer. This is the comprehensive treatment concept, it is possible to overcome cancer.

How to establish a comprehensive treatment concept of cancer?

The comprehensive treatment concept of cancer aims to study the clinical treatment of cancer from the biological characteristics of cancer cells and host body response in terms of both tumor and host.

(1) It is necessary to pay attention to a set of anti-cancer systems inherent in the human body, and should fully exert its immune system function, enhance immune surveillance, and prevent malignant cells from escaping.

(2) At the same time, radiotherapy and chemotherapy must also improve the immune function of the host. Cancer cells cannot rely solely on chemotherapy drugs, and must rely on the body's anti-cancer ability to eliminate cancer cells left by chemotherapy because of the limited ability of chemotherapy cytotoxic drugs to kill cancer cells.

1. **The duration of chemotherapy is limited and short-lived.** The time for chemotherapy to effectively kill cancer cells is only 1-5 days after intravenous injection. It has the effect of killing cancer cells, and then there is no effect of killing cancer cells. It is only a short time. Killing (1-5 days), cannot be "once and for all", after 5 days, the cancer cells continue to divide and proliferate. At the end of chemotherapy, the efficacy disappears, so it can only alleviate the improvement of a short period of several weeks, and must rely on the anti-cancer ability of the host immune function.

2. chemotherapy is a "double-edged sword", killing cancer cells also kills the host's bone marrow hematopoietic cells and promotes the decline of immune function. Therefore, chemotherapy must also protect, restore or enhance the host's immune function.

3. After radiotherapy and chemotherapy, the remaining cancer cells continue to divide, proliferate, and clone. It is still necessary to improve the anti-cancer ability of the host to inhibit the development of tumors for a long time.

Because radiotherapy and chemotherapy all contribute to the decline of immune function, the author proposes that radiotherapy or chemotherapy should be accompanied by immunotherapy and biological therapy. XZ-C immunomodulation anticancer Chinese medicine treatment must be reformed into immune + chemotherapy, immunity + radiotherapy.

(3) Improve the immune function of the host to inhibit the progression of the tumor. In the short-term, cancer treatment relies on chemotherapy drugs to kill cancer cells. In the long run, it depends on the host's immune function, and immune surveillance eliminates residual cancer cells. Therefore, the comprehensive treatment concept must improve the host's immune function through thymus protection and the immune function breast enhancement for the inhibition of tumor progression.

4

Principles of Cancer Treatment (Introduction)

The principle of cancer treatment - should change the concept and establish a comprehensive treatment concept

1. *Principles of cancer treatment – it should change the concept and establish a comprehensive treatment concept*
2. *the traditional therapy target is simple, only kill cancer cells*
3. *traditional therapy ignores the host's own resistance to cancer*
4. *Initiative to establish a comprehensive treatment perspective for both tumors and hosts*
5. *how to establish a comprehensive treatment concept of cancer*
6. *immune regulation is also the focus of comprehensive treatment of cancer*

The author believes that the treatment of cancer should overcome the current one-sided treatment concept that only targets cancer cells, and should change the concept and establish a comprehensive treatment concept. Because the process of cancer is the result of the mutual restriction of cancer cells and host function, the weakening of host anti-cancer power can lead to the occurrence and development of tumors. The enhanced anti-cancer power of the host can control the development of cancer. Rocker", this rise is falling. Therefore, treating cancer is not only to kill cancer cells, but also to protect the host, not to damage the host, enhance the host's anti-cancer power, and establish a comprehensive view of cancer treatment. *(Note: "Monograph" - "New Concepts and New Methods for Cancer Treatment" (the third monograph of Professor Xu Ze")*

1. the traditional therapy target is simple, just kill cancer cells

Traditional cancer therapy believes that cancer is the continuous division and proliferation of cells, so cancer cells are the culprit. The goal of cancer treatment must be to kill cancer cells. Radiotherapy and chemotherapy are all killing only cancer cells.

Why are traditional treatments that only kill cancer cells not reducing mortality? Why can't I stop recurrence and metastasis Why can only be relieved in the short term Why is it just relieved and not cured? Is it really because cancer can't be cured, or can it be cured without chemotherapy or chemotherapy alone? What are the problems, defects and drawbacks of radiotherapy and chemotherapy, or is there a problem with the medical strategy of killing only cancer cells? How many cancer cells did the patient kill each time he was hospitalized? How many cancer cells remain in the patient? Is the drug used in this chemotherapy sensitive? Is there resistance? These are not known exactly. However, this also suggests that traditional therapy does not conform to the actual situation of the biological characteristics of cancer cells. It only considers the aspect of killing cancer cells, but ignores the role of host function.

2. traditional therapy ignores the host's own resistance to cancer

In fact, the occurrence and development of tumor depends on the level of host immune function and the biological characteristics of the tumor itself, that is, the biological characteristics of the tumor cells and the host's influence on the constraints. If the two balance, then control; if the two is imbalance, the concer is progressing.

For nearly half a century, countries have been aiming at cancer cell tests and seeking drugs to kill cancer cells. The idea is to be affected by the antibiotic-bacterial mode and seek to kill cancer cells. I don't know if this is a completely different thing. Antibiotics only kill bacteria and do not kill normal cells, and can be used for drug susceptibility testing. The latter chemotherapeutic drugs kill both cancer cells and normal cells, and can not be used for drug susceptibility testing.

Traditional therapy only focuses on killing cancer cells, but ignores the host's own anti-cancer system and the body's own anti-cancer ability, ignoring the anti-cancer cells in the host (NK cell population, K cell population, LAK cell macrophage population, TK). Cell group), anti-cancer cell factor (IFN, IL-1, TNF), neglecting the role of tumor suppressor genes and tumor suppressor genes in the host (human cancer genes and tumor suppressor genes, also cancer metastasis genes) And the tumor suppressor gene), but also ignore the role of the neurohumoral system and endocrine hormones in the host. These influencing factors have important regulation, balance and stability effects on the host organism, and should be protected and activated against various anti-cancer factors in the human body.

3. Initiative to establish a comprehensive treatment perspective for both tumors and hosts

Since traditional therapies have not solved the problem in the true sense, it is necessary to establish a new treatment model to achieve better cancer treatment.

After deep thought and analysis, the author puts forward the concept of "balance theory" that affects the occurrence and development of cancer:

The biological characteristics of cancer

The restrictive ability of the host to cancer

Balance between the two controls

These two in balance , then control

these two imbalance, then progress

Therefore, the treatment target or target must target both the two sides: the tumor and the host.

Therapeutic target

The target of treatment

1.Host - immunity - **biology, cytokines, immune regulation, Chinese medicine**

2. cancer - cancer cells - **surgery, chemotherapy, radiotherapy**

The author believes that if the treatment target or target is only to kill cancer cells, it is only one aspect, which is unilateral or one-sided. If the treatment target or target is only immune regulation, it is only one aspect, and it is unilateral or one-sided. A one-sided treatment concept is impossible to overcome cancer. The treatment target should target both the host and the cancer, killing the cancer cells and protecting the host, enhancing immunity, protecting the chest from lifting, protecting the blood from the marrow, and enhancing the host's ability to fight cancer. This is the comprehensive treatment concept, and it is possible to overcome the cancer.

The author followed up more than 3,000 patients who had undergone surgery for extra- and extra-thoracic cancer. Most of the patients were found to have recurrence and metastasis within 2-3 years after surgery. After reviewing and reflecting on the experience and lessons of clinical oncology surgery for more than 50 years, I truly realized that to fight cancer not only to kill cancer cells, but also to inhibit tumors by increasing host anticancer power, the specific treatment goals are as follows:

(1) To control the occurrence and development of tumors, the host should first be considered, focusing on how to inhibit the occurrence and development of tumors by strengthening the anticancer power of the host.

(2) Strengthen the host's anti-cancer ability to inhibit tumor development, achieve tumor-bearing survival, and thus prolong survival. Try to make the host anti-cancer power strong enough to inhibit the tumor development for a long time, so as to achieve long-term tumor survival, only as a chronic disease.

4. how to establish a comprehensive treatment concept of cancer

The comprehensive treatment concept of cancer aims to study the clinical treatment of cancer from both the tumor and the host, from the biological characteristics of cancer cells and the host body reaction.

(1)   It is necessary to pay attention to a set of anti-cancer systems inherent in the human body, and should fully exert its immune system function, enhance immune surveillance, and prevent malignant cells from escaping. In fact, radiotherapy and chemotherapy can kill cancer cells. Due to the biological characteristics of cancer cells, the remaining cancer cells will continue to divide, proliferate and clone, which is multiplied by geometric progression, leading to cancer recurrence and metastasis.

(2)   Radiotherapy and chemotherapy must also improve the immune function of the host. Cancer cells can not rely solely on chemotherapy drugs, but must also rely on the body's anti-cancer ability to eliminate cancer cells left by chemotherapy because of the limited ability of chemotherapy cytotoxic drugs to kill cancer cells.

1.   Chemotherapy time is limited and short-lived, chemotherapy drugs can not be "once and for all", but the efficacy of killing cancer cells when intravenously taking chemotherapy drugs, the end of chemotherapy, the efficacy will disappear, even if it is done 4 times, 6 times, only It can be used for 2-3 months, and must rely on the host immune function to fight cancer.

2.   chemotherapy is a "double-edged sword". It kills cancer cells and also kills the host's bone marrow hematopoietic cells and immune cells, which promotes the decline of immune function. Therefore, chemotherapy must also restore or enhance the host's immune function.

3.   After radiotherapy and chemotherapy, the remaining tumor cells continue to divide, proliferate, and clone. It is still necessary to increase the anti-cancer ability of the host to inhibit tumor development for a long time.

Therefore, the author proposes that the current radiotherapy or chemotherapy should be simultaneously carried out immunotherapy, biological therapy, XZ-C immunomodulation anticancer Chinese medicine treatment, must be reformed into immune + chemotherapy, immune + radiotherapy.

(3)   Improve the immune function of the host to inhibit the progression of the tumor. In the short term, cancer treatment relies on chemotherapy drugs to kill cancer cells. In the long run, it depends on the host's immune function and immune surveillance to eliminate residual cancer cells. Therefore, the comprehensive treatment concept must improve the immune function of the host through chest enhancement, so as to inhibit the progression of the tumor.

Cancer is a systemic disease that should be studied from the biological characteristics and biological behavior of cancer and considering clinical treatment options. The immune system is particularly suitable for the removal of a small number of residual cancer cells, especially for quiescent tumor cells or stem cells that are difficult to kill by radiotherapy or chemotherapy, which helps to prolong the tumor-free survival of patients. Radiotherapy and chemotherapy can not kill all cancer cells, only a part of it can be killed. The remaining

cancer cells are destroyed by the immune cells of the host organism, so it is difficult to treat cancer by relying solely on radiotherapy and chemotherapy.

Tumor immunotherapy is an important part of tumor biotherapy and is the main points of the focus of comprehensive treatment. The theoretical basis of tumor biotherapy is that Oldham founded the theory of biological response regulation (BRM theory) in 1982. On this basis, it proposed four modality of cancer treatment in 1984. According to the BRM theory, under normal circumstances, the tumor is in a dynamic balance with the body's defense. The occurrence, invasion and metastasis of the tumor are completely caused by the imbalance of dynamic balance. If the condition that has been dysregulated is adjusted to a normal level, the growth of the tumor can be controlled and allowed to subside.

Biotherapy is to control tumor growth by adjusting, inducing or activating biologically active cells (or factors) with cytotoxic activity inherent in the BRM system in vivo to adjust the disorder. Biotherapy is different from traditional therapy in surgery, radiotherapy and chemotherapy. Tumor biotherapy mainly includes: (1) adoptive infusion of immune cells; (2) lymphokine/ cytokine application; (3) specific autoimmunity, including tumor vaccine Monoclonal antibody.

Under normal circumstances, the cell and humoral factors of the body's response system are in a delicate regulation. In the case of its imbalance, the body's response or response ability will be significantly affected. The use of biological response modifiers is to make the balance unbalanced. The state of the body can be restored to a normal state to achieve the purpose of preventing and treating tumors.

The biological response modifier regulates the immune function of the body and restores the immune system function of the suppressed body. These drugs exert their regulatory functions by activating the body's immune system, with more microorganisms and plant sources.

5. immune regulation and control treatment is the focus of comprehensive treatment of cancer

After 4 years of experimental research and 16 years of clinical validation, XZ-C immunomodulation anticancer Chinese medicine is a BRM-like drug that has been screened from natural drug resources.

XZ-C immunomodulation anticancer traditional Chinese medicine was experimentally screened from 200 kinds of traditional Chinese medicines by the author's laboratory. Firstly, 200 kinds of traditional Chinese medicines were screened by in vitro culture of cancer cells, and direct damage of cancer cells in culture tubes was observed. The chemotherapeutic drug cyclophosphamide and normal cells cultured in vitro were used as a control group to compare the tumor inhibition rates. As a result, a batch of traditional Chinese medicines with a certain tumor inhibition rate for cancer cell proliferation were selected. Then, the tumor-bearing animal model was further made, and the in vivo anti-tumor screening test of the tumor-bearing animal model was carried out on 200 kinds of Chinese medicines, and analyzed and evaluated by scientific, objective and rigorous screening. The experimental results show that only 48 kinds of traditional Chinese medicines have a good tumor inhibition rate.

The application principle of XZ-C immunomodulation Chinese medicine:

XZ-C immunomodulatory anticancer Chinese medicine with BRM and BRM-like effects can enhance the body's immune response and strengthen the body's tumor immune surveillance. When the cells are mutated or the tumor is very small, the effect is better. Through surgery or radiation therapy, drug treatment works best when the tumor is minimized.

For those who have lost the opportunity for surgery, poor physical fitness, can not tolerate radiotherapy, chemotherapy, immunotherapy has a certain effect, can reduce the symptoms of patients and prolong the survival time of patients.

After radical resection of the tumor, in order to reduce recurrence and metastasis, XZ-C immunomodulation can be used to treat anticancer Chinese medicine. After surgical resection of large tumors, it is also feasible to eliminate cancer cells that may remain and distant cancer cells. -C immunomodulation Chinese medicine treatment.

If the tumor can not be removed, radiotherapy or chemotherapy can be used first to kill the tumor cells in a large amount, so that the tumor burden in the body is reduced, and then XZ-C immunomodulation is used to treat the Chinese medicine.

In short, in the case of a healthy immune system, the body can limit and eliminate tumors through its cellular and humoral immune responses. The growing tumor has many effects on the body's immune system, which can inhibit the immune function of the body and promote the development of the tumor.

Therefore, the treatment of cancer must target both the host and the tumor. It is necessary to use theory to guide the clinical, and at the same time to treat cancer cells and host anticancer power, and establish a comprehensive treatment concept.

(5) Cancer treatment model (introduction)

Cancer treatment requires a scientifically designed treatment plan. The occurrence of cancer is the balance between the body's immune and anti-cancer ability and tumor development, the loss of immune surveillance, and the further development of the tumor. The treatment must restore balance and stability.

Cancer treatment requires a "multidisciplinary comprehensive treatment plan". This program is an organic comprehensive treatment that must meet the actual conditions of the patient's condition.

The combination of multidisciplinary comprehensive treatment must have a reasonable theoretical basis, must be a comprehensive treatment concept, and the host's new understanding of tumor progression and metastasis has important theoretical value and clinical guiding significance. In the formulation of anti-cancer invasion and anti-metastatic programs, we should consider the rational combination of disciplines, methods, techniques and drugs from the perspective of tumor and host.

Based on the above analysis, in the diagnosis, treatment, drug development, anti-cancer and anti-metastasis strategies should be considered from the perspective of both tumor and host. This may be a fundamental change in the current one-sided treatment plan to kill only cancer cells, and then establish the principle of comprehensive treatment.

How to combine multidisciplinary treatment? The author believes that, first of all, we should change our mindset, update our thinking, establish a comprehensive treatment concept of cancer, and arrange intervention, regulation and treatment measures throughout the whole process of cancer occurrence, development, recurrence and metastasis. The main treatment methods commonly used in various disciplines are based on full-course treatment and short-course treatment, comprehensive division of labor, and organic cooperation.

1 full treatment. Radical surgery is the main treatment, the tumor has been resected, the lymph nodes have been cleaned, and then long-term or full-course biological treatment, immunotherapy, cytokines, gene therapy, XZ-C immunomodulation anticancer Chinese medicine treatment, Chinese and Western combined immunomodulation Chinese medicine treatment To enhance the host's anti-cancer immunity, regulate or control recurrence and metastasis. It can be used throughout the treatment of cancer.

2 short-course treatment. With radiotherapy and chemotherapy as the mainstay, it can only be treated intermittently, or short-range

assault to kill cancer cells, instead of not being able to treat the whole course or long course of treatment, nor can it be "once and for all", because it takes 3-5 days to kill cancer cells. The effect is not to kill cancer cells. After short-term remission, the cancer cells continue to divide, proliferate, recur, and metastasize. Because they can kill cancer cells only for 4 cycles or 6 cycles, drug resistance may occur over a long period of time.

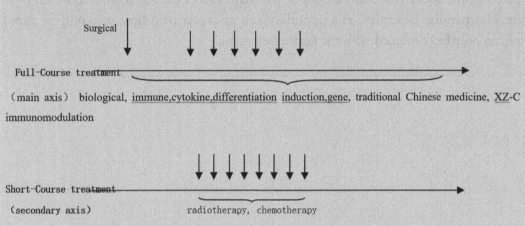

Multidisciplinary comprehensive treatment combination mode

The above strategies for full-course treatment and short-course treatment are considered from the perspective of both tumor and host, which may fundamentally change the one-sided treatment concept of killing cancer cells.

Short-course treatment is only a short-term stage in the overall course of cancer patients, so it should be adjuvant therapy (or pseudo-axis) because it only targets unilateral cancer cells. Do not travel long distances, not excessive.

Traditional radiotherapy and chemotherapy are only for the tumor, which is limited, one-sided, not comprehensive, and thus it is difficult to overcome cancer. Because the process of cancer is the result of regulatory imbalances, both host and tumor factors must be addressed, and the host's response determines the final outcome. The cure should be through regulation rather than single killing.

The whole process of treatment is the whole process of cancer from the occurrence, development, recurrence, metastasis and progression of the disease. It is aimed at the tumor and the host. The radical resection of the carcinogen is based on biotherapy, immunotherapy, gene therapy and cytokines. Treatment, XZ-C immunomodulation and other traditional Chinese medicine treatment to improve the host's anti-cancer power, this scientific and comprehensive comprehensive treatment is reasonable and scientific, in line with the pathogenesis of cancer, pathophysiology, in line with the biological characteristics of cancer cells And biological behavior, therefore, it can overcome cancer.

Therefore, the whole treatment should be the main axis of cancer treatment, which is the cure. Short-course treatment, as a secondary axis of cancer treatment, can only be cured, and can only be combined with the entire treatment.

5

Cancer treatment mode (introduction)

—A new model for the combination of multidisciplinary treatment of cancer

1. Why is there a new model for organic comprehensive treatment?
2. How to formulate a new multi-disciplinary organic comprehensive treatment model
3. Initiatives for specific programs for multidisciplinary treatment of cancer

The author believes that the combination of multidisciplinary comprehensive treatment must have a reasonable theoretical basis, and the host's new understanding of tumor progression and metastasis has important theoretical value and clinical guiding significance. Before formulating anti-cancer, anti-metastatic strategies and comprehensive treatment plans, we should rationally consider the disciplines, methods, techniques, and drugs with theoretical basis from the perspective of tumor and host, and integrate these organics. This is the comprehensive treatment concept. Note: "Monograph" - is the series of monographs by the author Xu Ze (XU ZE), the first of the following articles: quoted from the "Monograph" original text, are the same.

In the 21st century, the treatment of cancer has entered the era of multidisciplinary treatment.

At present, the status quo of comprehensive treatment is based on the traditional three major treatment methods. How to apply other comprehensive treatment methods depends on the first consultation department. Most patients are diagnosed with chemotherapy for the first time, so they are treated with chemotherapy and chemotherapy. If the patient is in the first radiotherapy department, then radiotherapy followed by chemotherapy. If the first diagnosis is surgery and there is a surgical indication, the operation is first, and then chemotherapy or radiotherapy is performed. If there is no indication for surgery, radiotherapy and chemotherapy are performed. As a result of this comprehensive treatment, there are still many patients with recurrence, metastasis, and even some patients have immune failure.

Biological therapy, immunotherapy, differentiation therapy, cytokine therapy, and integrated immunotherapy with integrated Chinese and Western medicine have not been included in the treatment of most oncologists.

Authors: Xu Ze (China) ; Xu Jie(China) ; Bin Wu(America)

1. Why should we propose a new model of organic comprehensive treatment?

Research in cancer therapy must be based on tumor biology, and the two must be consistent. Tumor biology has evolved into molecular biology, cytokines, and gene levels, and the theoretical basis of traditional cancer therapies still remains at the cellular level half a century ago. In the past 10 years, the research trends and clinical application status of anti-tumor drugs at home and abroad have shown that traditional anti-tumor drugs have more and more clinical applications due to their adverse reactions, poor targeting and easy tolerance of tumors to drugs. limits. It can be considered that anticancer drug research has developed to a new stage, and will face the update of theory, technology and ideas. Traditional therapies, traditional ideas and working methods based on the cytotoxic drugs to kill cancer cells are being affected.

Since the 1980s, medical molecular science, molecular immunology, immunopharmacology, traditional Chinese medicine immunopharmacology, and cytokines have developed rapidly, and new biotherapeutics have emerged to promote the development of cancer therapeutics. Biotherapy, immunotherapy, differentiation inducers, biological response modifiers, and molecular-level Chinese and Western medicine combined with immunomodulatory Chinese medicine are on the stage. In recent years, the development of new tumor vaccines and gene therapy have provided attractive prospects for cancer treatment.

The author believes that cancer treatment requires a scientifically designed treatment plan. The occurrence of cancer is the balance between the body's immune and anti-cancer ability and tumor development. It loses the immune surveillance and further develops the tumor. The treatment must make both Restore balance and stability.

2. How to formulate a multidisciplinary organic comprehensive treatment plan

    (1) The treatment of cancer requires a "multidisciplinary organic comprehensive treatment plan". This program is organic and comprehensive treatment, and must be in line with the actual situation of the patient's condition:

        1. The biological characteristics of cancer cells are that after the malignant cells in the body become cancer cells, they continue to undergo sexual division, proliferation, cloning, and throughout the whole process of cancer development, development, metastasis, and recurrence, so the treatment measures must be controlled accordingly. Treatment is carried out throughout the process, not just at a certain stage of the disease.

        2. Cancer is a development process, cancer cells are characterized by uncontrolled infinite reproduction, and the malignant process is the result of imbalance. The tumor maintains a certain relationship with the host, and the host's response determines the final result.

        3. According to the biological behavior of cancer cells, the multi-step and multi-step of cancer cell metastasis, the eight-step, three-stage and two-point line of cancer

cell transfer, intervene and block the cancer cells on the way of metastasis, adopt a scientific organic combination A new model of treatment.

(2) The combination of multidisciplinary comprehensive treatment must have a reasonable theoretical basis. It must be a comprehensive treatment concept, a new understanding of the host's influence on tumor progression and metastasis, and it has important theoretical value and clinical guiding significance. When formulating anti-cancer invasion and anti-metastatic programs, we should consider from the two perspectives of tumor and host, and organically integrate which reasonable theoretically based disciplines, methods, techniques and drugs.

What are the most important determinants of cancer development, development and metastasis? Is it a host or a tumor? Is the host's immune anti-cancer ability, or the invasion and metastasis of cancer cells? In the past half century, research has focused on cancer cells themselves, and countries are targeting how to kill cancer cells. Therefore, although the traditional treatment of killing only cancer cells has made some remarkable progress, they have not solved the problem fundamentally, but only the symptoms are not cured.

In recent years, people have turned more attention to host factors, through the experimental study of the etiology, pathogenesis, pathophysiology and cancer invasion and metastasis mechanism of cancer, to explore the interaction between host anti-cancer immunity and tumor, and to find the right The regulatory mechanism of cancer cell invasion and metastasis. Therefore, the author proposes the concept of "balance", that is, cancer is the balance between the biological characteristics of cancer cells and the host's immune and anti-cancer power. If balance is restored, cancer control and treatment must be targeted to the host and Two aspects of the tumor restore balance and stability.

The experimental study of the interaction and relationship between the host and the tumor and the analysis of clinical practice experience and lessons are whether cancer cells or host factors determine the occurrence, development, metastasis and recurrence of cancer. What is the cause of cancer death? Why does cancer cause death? We have recognized that the main cause of death in cancer patients is metastasis and recurrence, but how does recurrence and metastasis lead to death? Our initial analysis, thinking, and experience are due to complications and immune failure, and this final result should be considered as both the tumor itself and the host factor.

The immune function of the host is low. The cell malignant → most of the cells are engulfed by the body's immune system. The residual malignant cells continue to divide, proliferate, clone, and form tumor metastasis.

The author believes that it is the interaction between cancer cells and the host microenvironment and immune anti-cancer power, which ultimately determines the progress of cancer, whether metastases can form and when. The revelation of this interaction regulation mechanism has important theoretical value and clinical guiding significance. In formulating anti-cancer anti-metastasis strategies and new drug development, we should consider from the perspective of tumor factors and host factors, and find effective for us. The intervention method and the development of new drugs provide a theoretical basis. The XZ-C immunomodulation anticancer Chinese medicine developed by us is the theoretical basis and experimental basis for breast enhancement and bone marrow protection from the enhancement of host factors.

Based on the above analysis, in the diagnosis, treatment, drug development, formulation of anti-cancer and anti-metastasis strategies, should be considered from the perspective of both tumor and host. This may be a fundamental change in the current one-sided treatment plan to kill only cancer cells, and then establish the principle of comprehensive treatment.

3. Initiatives for specific programs for multidisciplinary treatment of cancer

How to combine multidisciplinary treatment? The author believes that, first of all, we should change our concepts and update our thinking, establish a comprehensive treatment concept of cancer, and arrange intervention, regulation and treatment measures throughout the whole process of cancer occurrence, development, recurrence and metastasis. The main treatment methods commonly used in various disciplines are based on full-course treatment or short-course treatment, with comprehensive division of labor and organic cooperation (below).

(1) full treatment

Radical surgery is the main treatment, the tumor has been resected, the lymph nodes have been cleaned, and then long-term or full-course biological treatment, immunotherapy, cytokine therapy, differentiation induction therapy, gene therapy, Chinese and Western combined immunotherapy, XZ-C immunomodulation Anti-cancer Chinese medicine treatment to enhance the host's anti-cancer immunity, regulate or control recurrence and metastasis. They can be used throughout the treatment of cancer diseases.

(2) short-course treatment

Mainly for radiotherapy and chemotherapy, it is staged treatment or intermittent treatment, or short-range assault to kill cancer cells, instead of not being able to treat the whole course or long course of treatment, nor can it be "once and for all", because it can only kill 4 cycles or 6 cancer cells cycles may be resistant for a long time.

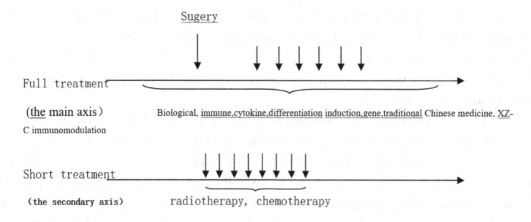

Figure Multidisciplinary treatment combination model diagram

The above strategies for full-course treatment and short-course treatment are considered from the perspective of tumor factors and host, which may fundamentally change the one-sided treatment concept of killing cancer cells.

Short-course treatment is only a short-term stage in the overall course of cancer patients, so it should be adjuvant therapy (or called the secondary axis) because it only targets unilateral cancer cells.

1. Biological characteristics of cancer cells: The formation of cancer originates from the malignant transformation of single cells. Cancer cells undergo progressive division and proliferation. Cancer is a development process, not a form or entity. Therefore, it tries its best to kill cancer cells. It is also impossible to kill cancer cells. As long as there are cancer cells remaining, they will continue, continue to divide, proliferate, and relapse. Moreover, chemotherapy can not kill cancer stem cells. Cancer stem cells must continue to divide and proliferate, forming cancer cells. Therefore, the treatment of cancer cells only does not conform to the biological characteristics and biological behavior of cancer cells.

2. The effective time of cytotoxicity killing is time-limited, only effective when used, and it is invalid after the passage of time, and can not be "once and for all". Its action time is limited, and the remaining 10^6-10^7 cancer cells will eventually be destroyed by the host body's immunity. Moreover, the cancer stem cells continue to form cancer cells, so the radiotherapy and chemotherapy can only be relieved for several months and cannot be cured.

3. chemotherapy to kill cancer cells is only a first-order kinetics, its lethality is limited, it can only kill 10^6-10^7 cancer cells.

4. chemotherapeutic drugs are "double-edged swords", which kills cancer cells and kills normal cells, bone marrow hematopoietic cells and immune cells, causing a decline in host immune function.

Traditional radiotherapy and chemotherapy are only factors that target cancer cells. They are limited, one-sided, and not comprehensive, making it difficult to overcome cancer. Because the process of carcinogenesis is the result of regulatory imbalances, both host and tumor factors must be addressed, and the host's response determines the final outcome. The cure should be through regulation rather than single killing.

(3) The whole process of treatment is from the occurrence, development, recurrence, metastasis and progress of cancer. It is the two factors of tumor and host. It is radically resected for the carcinogen, and it is treated with biological therapy, immunotherapy and gene therapy. Cytokines, immune regulation and other traditional Chinese medicines improve the anti-cancer power of the host organism. This scientific and comprehensive comprehensive treatment concept is reasonable and scientific, in line with the pathogenesis and pathophysiology of cancer, and conforms to the biological characteristics and biology of cancer cells. Behavior, so it is also possible to overcome cancer.

Therefore, the whole treatment should be the main axis of cancer treatment, mainly based on surgical treatment, while biotherapy, immune regulation treatment, cytokine therapy, gene therapy, differentiation induction therapy, and Chinese medicine immunomodulation therapy are applied throughout the whole process of cancer treatment. This is the way to cure the problem. Short-course treatment should be the secondary axis of cancer treatment, mainly radiotherapy and chemotherapy, and cooperate with the whole treatment.

The author believes that the above-mentioned combination of multidisciplinary comprehensive treatment has a reasonable theoretical guidance and is in line with the actual condition of the patient's condition, which is reasonable and scientific.

After half a century of clinical case treatment experience and lessons learned, single cancer killing, can not control cancer, can not beat cancer, is a one-sided treatment, not comprehensive.

The target or target of cancer treatment should be directed at both the host and the tumor. Which one is the main one, who decides the final fate of the cancer patient, should also be the tumor and the host.

It is necessary to update ideas, change concepts, and establish a comprehensive concept of cancer treatment in the whole process of cancer occurrence, development, recurrence, and metastasis.

A new treatment mode of "spindle + secondary shaft" should be established, which will be a reasonable and scientific design, both theoretically guided and in line with the actual condition.

It must be people-oriented, eliminate the adverse reactions of radiotherapy and chemotherapy as much as possible, and improve the safety of patients. Every drug and every technology must accurately understand its toxicity and safety to ensure a reasonable theoretical basis to guide the clinical.

In short, the treatment of cancer, whether early, middle or late, requires multidisciplinary treatment. There must be reasonable theory to guide the clinical.

In the past 20 years, there have been many reports on the treatment of cancer by traditional Chinese medicine, and its prospects have attracted much attention. Especially with the deepening of medical and immunological research, people have realized that the disorder of the body's immune system is closely related to the occurrence and development of tumors. Traditional Chinese medicine has its unique characteristics and advantages by adjusting the body's immune function to treat tumors. The immunomodulatory effects of traditional Chinese medicine and the development of traditional Chinese medicine immunomodulatory drugs will be valued and favored all over the world. XZ-C immunoregulation of traditional Chinese medicine combined with surgery, radiotherapy and chemotherapy can fully exert its immune regulation in the course of treatment, significantly prolong the survival of patients, improve the quality of life of patients, and reflect the characteristics and advantages of traditional Chinese medicine in treating cancer, but The weakness is that the change in the tumor itself is not very significant.

Because the above various methods have their own characteristics and effects on the treatment of cancer, the curative effects are not the same, and each has its own weaknesses. This requires the advantages and disadvantages of various therapies, and the gains and losses of patients. Measure, what is the strength and weakness of the treatment, what will the patient get and lose? These treatments should be long, complementary, short, organically and reasonably combined to form a comprehensive treatment for cancer, so as to significantly reduce adverse drug reactions, improve the quality of life of patients, and prolong the patient's Overall survival. In the past 34 years, the author has practiced the comprehensive treatment of more than 12,000 patients with advanced cancer using surgery + XZ-C immunomodulation and anti-cancer traditional Chinese medicine. Most of the results obtained the effects of improving quality of life, stabilizing lesions, controlling metastasis, living with tumors, and significantly prolonging life.

Quoted from the "Monograph" original Chapter 4

6

Principles of cancer metastasis treatment (introduction)

1. *cancer research or conquering cancer, the key is anti-metastasis*
2. *the basic principle of cancer treatment is anti-metastasis*
3. *The main feature of the new concept of cancer treatment, namely control transfer*
4. *One of the goals of 21st century cancer treatment should be anti-metastasis*
5. *"If it didn't research or study cancer metastasis, improving the efficacy would be an empty talk."*

From the clinical practice of nearly one hundred years, it can be seen that the traditional three major therapies: surgery, radiotherapy, chemotherapy for malignant tumors have achieved good results, and many patients have significantly reduced tumors after radiotherapy and chemotherapy.

But soon after, the tumor recurred, enlarged, and metastasized.

The author summarizes the experience and lessons of both positive and negative clinical practice cases over the past 60 years. Combined with long-term experimental research and clinical practice experience, the author has the following new understandings, and proposes new theoretical concepts and advocates the implementation of new treatment strategies.

1. cancer research or conquering cancer, the key is anti-metastasis

Metastasis is the leading cause of cancer death, so metastasis is the key to cancer treatment.

Since the 20th century, the goal of cancer treatment has been to kill cancer cells in primary and metastatic cancers. Although after a century of hard work, the mortality rate of cancer still accounts for the first place in human disease mortality. **The main cause of such a high case fatality rate is the transfer. The original traditional treatment failed to reduce the long-term high mortality rate. The main reason for the failure was the failure to target metastasis and control metastasis.**

Today, the main problem with cancer treatment is how to resist metastasis. If the problem of cancer metastasis cannot be solved, cancer treatment cannot be advanced. Therefore, one of the goals of 21 cancer treatment should be anti-metastasis.

Recognizing the above issues prompts us to update our thinking, change our mindset, and find new ways to resist metastasis and overcome cancer. To this end, the author proposes that according to the biological characteristics of cancer and the biological behavior of cancer metastasis, analyze and understand the host immune status, multi-step and multi-link of cancer metastasis, molecular transfer mechanism, etc., and propose a new treatment mode for anti-cancer metastasis.

Academician Tang Yuxian from the Institute of Liver Cancer of Fudan University, in the article "I see cancer clinical research" on November 9, 2007, said: **"To improve efficacy is an empty talk not to research cancer metastasis."**

Internationally, research on tumor metastasis has been highly valued since the 1990s. The Metastasis Research Society was established and the journal Clinical and Experimental Metastasis was published. Cancer metastasis was also established in Tokyo, Japan. Research.

The study of domestic transfer started late. In 1996, Professor Gao Jin published "Invasion and Metastasis of Cancer - Basic Research and Clinical", the first monograph on cancer metastasis in China. In 2003, Academician Tang Wei published the book "Basic and Clinical of Liver Cancer Metastasis and Recurrence". In the monograph, it puts forward: **"The next important goal of primary liver cancer research - prevention and treatment of recurrence and metastasis", " "Metastasis and recurrence have become a bottleneck for further improving the survival rate of liver cancer, and one of the most important difficulties in conquering cancer."** These academic monographs have promoted the importance of domestic scholars on tumor metastasis research. In 2006, Professor Xu Ze published the book "New Concepts and New Methods for Cancer Metastasis Treatment" and proposed some related theories.

2. **the basic principle of cancer treatment is anti-metastasis**

(1) **The biological behavior of cancer cells, that is, the unique behavior of invasion and metastasis. Metastasis is a malignant behavior. It is well known that the fundamental difference between a benign tumor and a malignant tumor is that the former does not transfer but the latter shifts**. If there is a way to prevent cancer cells from metastasizing, then malignant tumors may become benign tumors. **85%-95% of cancer patients die from metastasis. Most patients will not die if no metastasis occurs. If cancer didn't metastasis or cancer metastasis could be controlled well, the cancer will become** less scary. Therefore, the principle of cancer treatment should be the development of anti-metastatic treatment programs and intervention programs, the development of anti-metastatic drugs, the design of cancer cells in the metastasis, and the multi-step, multi-step, multi-factor and multi-transfer one or several links in the gene are truncated or blocked to achieve controlled transfer.

(2)   How to resist the transfer. The biological characteristics and biological behavior of cancer cells are invasion and metastasis. The reason why cancer is malignant is that it is caused by extensive invasion and metastasis. For more than a century, the traditional three major treatment targets are mainly for primary cancer and metastatic cancer, surgical removal of primary cancer mass or treatment of metastatic cancer with radiotherapy and other local treatments. It is generally believed that the primary cancerous mass and the metastatic cancerous mass are visible or tangible, which is a local problem and can be treated by surgery or radiotherapy. Reviewing and reflecting on the author's clinical practice for more than 60 years is also based on the above-mentioned understanding, and has carried out many "radiation cures" of various cancers in the chest and abdomen. However, in 1985, the authors followed up on 3,000 patients who had undergone surgery after surgery, and suddenly realized that How to prevent postoperative recurrence and metastasis is the core issue that determines the long-term efficacy of cancer. Primary cancer or metastatic cancer may be localized, while distant metastasis is a systemic problem.

Since the 1970s, in view of the recurrence and metastasis rate after cancer surgery, postoperative series of adjuvant chemotherapy has been used to control postoperative recurrence, and even chemotherapy has been started before surgery (such as breast cancer), but the results are not satisfactory. In many patients, postoperative adjuvant chemotherapy failed to prevent recurrence and metastasis, and in some cases, immune chemotherapy was induced by intensive chemotherapy. These are worthy of clinical doctors should seriously, calmly think, review, analyze, reflect, cancer treatment focus should also turn to how to prevent recurrence, anti-metastasis.

In the past 20 years, the understanding of the mechanism of molecular metastasis of cancer has made great progress, and there is still no good law at home and abroad for anti-cancer cell metastasis. Although many new anticancer drugs have appeared in recent years, the efficacy has not been satisfactorily improved. The reason why some advanced cancer surgery can not cure radical resection is the distant metastasis of lymph nodes. Therefore, inhibiting cancer metastasis is the key to reducing cancer mortality and improving efficacy.

The goal of traditional therapy is relatively simple, only to kill cancer cells, which is not all in line with the actual situation of cancer biological characteristics. Such as cancer cell invasion behavior, metastasis and multiple steps, the molecular biological mechanism of metastasis, the body's immune response and the cause of recurrence. At present, people have realized that anticancer drugs do not necessarily resist metastasis, and anti-metastatic drugs may not kill cancer cells.

Therefore, the author believes that the key to current cancer research is anti-metastasis. Studying how to resist metastasis is the core issue of cancer treatment.

3. The main feature of the new concept of cancer treatment, namely control metastasis

Killing cancer cells in the human body should rely on two kinds of forces: one is the external force of surgery, radiotherapy, and chemotherapy; the other is the internal strength of the patient's own immunity. Drugs, surgery, and various treatment techniques are important for the treatment of patients, but the body's own immunity is more important. Many problems must be solved by the patient's own strength, such as nutritional problems. Although a sufficient amount of nutrients are given, if the patient's body can not be absorbed and utilized, it is difficult to achieve the purpose, and if the incision is healed, it must rely on the patient's own healing. Function, external factors can only affect or promote its healing.

The body's own immunity can kill cancer cells. According to literature, a small tumor (1-8g) can release millions and tens of millions of cancer cells into the bloodstream within 24 hours, but the human immune system can put the vast majority of blood (99.9). %) Cancer cells kill, and less than 0.1% of cancer cells survive and continue to grow into metastatic cancer. **The author's experimental data show that 10^5 S-180 malignant cells were injected into the tail vein of Kunming mice. After 24 hours, the mice could eliminate 99% of the cancer cells by their own immunity. Oral administration of XZ-C1 and XZ-C4 immunomodulatory Chinese medicine to mice can eliminate more cancer cells. In the past 10 years, according to the clinical data of the anti-cancer metastasis research room of Wuhan Shuguang Oncology Clinic, the routine use of XZ-C1 and XZ-C4 in patients can indeed eliminate a certain amount of cancer cells in the process of metastasis**.

The human body has a certain anti-cancer ability, because the human body has a complete anti-cancer system, such as anti-cancer cell population (NK cell population, K cell population, LAK cell population, macrophage population, TK cell population), anticancer effect, anticancer effect of anti-cancer cell factor system (IFN, IL-2, TNF, LT), role of tumor suppressor gene and tumor suppressor gene, and role of neurohumoral and endocrine hormones. These anti-cancer systems and their effects in the human body play a role in regulating, balancing, and stabilizing the anti-cancer function of the body. Therefore, it must be protected, activated, and mobilized.

The occurrence, development, and metastasis of cancer are closely related to the decline of immune function. Cancer can directly invade immune organs and cause immune function decline or inhibition. It can also release immunosuppressive factors to reduce host immunity or induce inhibitory cell growth in vivo. When a cancer occurs, the host thymus has been inhibited, and chemotherapy inhibits the bone marrow, which is like "adding frost." Traditional therapy ignores the body's own anti-cancer ability, neglects the anti-cancer power of anti-cancer cells, anti-cancer factors and anti-transfer genes in the host, so that the entire central immune organ is damaged and cannot be effectively protected. This is traditional therapy. This is the reason why the effect cannot be improved.

The author believes that in cancer treatment, attention must be paid to the power of exerting and relying on the host's own anti-cancer system.

The main feature of the new concept of cancer treatment is to control the transfer and protect the patient's immunity, rather than simply killing cancer cells.

7

New concept of cancer metastasis treatment (introduction)

- Targeting or aiming cancer cells on the way to metastasis

1. *The main manifestations of cancer in the human body or the main existing form of cancer in the human body*
2. *Traditional cancer therapies believe that there are two forms*
3. *The new concept of cancer treatment is considered to have three forms.*
4. *The third form of research and understanding process of cancer in human body*
5. *The research and understanding of the third form of cancer in the human body*
6. *the goal of cancer treatment should be directed to the above three forms of existence*
7. *To target or aim cancer cells on the way will bring a new dawn for conquering cancer or the fight against cancer*

The author has carried out more than 60 years of clinical experience in oncology surgery and more than 10 years of laboratory research results, carefully analyzed and summarized, and formed a unique new understanding and new concept of cancer metastasis, and proposed new technologies and new methods of cancer anti-metastasis treatment. The main contents include: 1 three manifestations of cancer in the human body; 2 "two points and one line" theory of the whole process of cancer development; 3 "eight steps and three stages" of cancer metastasis; 4 human anti-cancer metastasis treatment The third field; 5 cancer metastasis treatment "three steps"; 6 independently developed XZ-C immune regulation anti-cancer series of traditional Chinese medicine preparations.

The following new understandings, new doctrines, and new concepts have not been mentioned in the literature and textbooks so far. They are all the lessons learned by the author after half a century of clinical practice and translated into theory after more than 60 years of experimental research analysis, reflection, and enlightenment. These theoretical innovations have also become the theoretical system of the new concept of cancer anti-metastasis treatment, which is unique to the author. It has independent intellectual property rights of independent innovation and original innovation.

1. Traditional cancer therapies believe that there are two forms

Traditional cancer therapies believe that the presence of cancer in humans has two manifestations: one is the primary tumor mass of the primary tumor, and the other is metastatic nodules or metastases.

The therapeutic goals or targets of traditional cancer therapies are directed at both manifestations, ie, for primary tumors and metastatic tumors. Because both primary tumors and metastatic tumors are composed of cancer cells, and the therapeutic goal is to kill cancer cells. Traditional therapy relies mainly on surgery, radiotherapy, and chemotherapy to achieve this goal.

The main reasons for the failure of traditional therapy treatment are recurrence and metastasis.

2. The new concept of cancer treatment is considered to have three forms.

At the international conference, the author first published a new theoretical understanding that the third form of cancer in the human body is the cancer cell group on the way to transfer.

The new concept of cancer metastasis treatment believes that there are three manifestations of cancer in the human body: the first is primary cancer; the second is metastatic cancer; the third is cancer cell group on the way to metastasis.

It is these cancer cell populations on the way to metastasis that may be the main cause of recurrence and metastasis after cancer surgery.

The cancer cells on the way to metastasis are invisible to the naked eye during surgery. For example, when performing "radical gastrectomy", the gastric cancer mass and the metastatic lymph nodes can be seen, but whether there are cancer cells in the bloodstream of the stomach vein and the portal vein or not and how many cancer cells is inside are invisible. Where did the cancer cells in these venous bloodstreams have already reached? Whether had these groups of cancer cells that are squeezed into the venous blood flow by the touch of surgery reached the gastric vein or reached the hepatic portal vein, and even reached the intrahepatic portal vein branch? **During surgery exploration and removal of gastric cancer masses and lymph node dissection, it is impossible to not touch the cancer mass, because of the operation of the hand it will inevitably cause a large number of cancer cells to be squeezed off, and a large amount of tumor veins flow into the blood circulation and flow into the hepatic portal vein. However, the surgeon is not visible.** These cancer cells that flow into the hepatic portal vein flow to the intrahepatic portal vein. Usually, various immune cells in the portal vein are immunologically monitored for cancer cells entering the blood circulation of the hepatic portal vein, and are subjected to phagocytosis and to kill all of them. However, **in a short period of time**, the immune cells of the portal vein system cannot treat these sudden influx of cancer cells. After some time, some cancer cells escaped from immunosurveillance, and cancer cells that survived the blood flow may be implanted in the hepatic sinus, generating blood vessels and forming intrahepatic metastases.

This is a phenomenon and a fact, but it has not been thought of or discovered in the past. This is a dynamic form of cancer cells in the human body. The author's Institute of Experimental

Authors: Xu Ze (China) ; Xu Jie(China) ; Bin Wu(America)

Surgery, Cancer Research and Recurrence Research Laboratory, through the analysis and research of more than 10,000 outpatients with cancer metastasis, found that the essence of metastasis is the cancer cells during metastasis, the goal of anti-metastasis and the treatment" The target should be directed to the cancer cells on the way to metastasis, that is, the third form of cancer in the human body. Since this has not been recognized in the past, it is only for the treatment of primary and metastatic cancer, and tries to reduce or eliminate it. I don't know if the tumor shrinks and does not mean that it does not transfer. The long-term efficacy of traditional therapy often fails due to recurrence and metastasis. This suggests that the lack of understanding in traditional therapeutics has led to the failure of its long-term efficacy.

3. Research and understanding process of cancer in the third manifestation of human body

(1) **Where are the cancer cells on the way of metastasis?**
Since we have realized that the key to cancer treatment is anti-metastatic, how can we resist metastasis? How can we understand the specific processes, steps and mechanisms of cancer cell metastasis? Just like fighting an enemy, how many enemies should you find? where is it? What is the trend? How do these cancer cells move? What is the law of its activities? Where are the cancer cells in the process of metastasis? Which or which links should be blocked or blocked? How should the goal of combating cancer metastasis be embodied?

(2) Experimental study on tracking the fate and regularity of cancer cells on the way to transfer

In order to solve the above series of problems, we must carry out experimental basic research on cancer, perform cancer cell transplantation, establish a tumor animal model, and carry out a series of experimental tumor research: 1 to explore the mechanism and law of cancer invasion and metastasis; 2 to explore tumor and immunity, Immune organs, and the relationship between immune organs and tumors; 3 looking for effective measures to regulate cancer invasion and metastasis. The author's laboratory spent more than three years conducting experimental studies on animal models of cancer metastasis, **as well as experimental observations to track the fate and regularity of cancer cells during metastasis.**

In the animal experiment, 10^5 cancer cells were injected intravenously from the mice, and no cancer cells were detected in the blood after 48 hours. So who killed these injected cancer cells? The analysis speculates that some cells may be destroyed after being injected into the circulatory system, which are not adapted to the environment, damaged by blood flow or blocked by the microcirculation, but most of the cancer cells that enter the blood circulation are mainly the immunity of the mice themselves. That is, a large number of immune cells in the blood circulation of mice are eliminated by phagocytosis. Therefore, in the anti-metastatic treatment, cancer cells and cancer cell groups in the process of treatment must protect the immunity of the host organism, and should try to mobilize, restore, and activate the immune function of the immune system, and should not or try to avoid hitting or damage. Reduce host immunity and immune system function. How to protect, mobilize, and activate the host's immune function to cope with cancer cells on the way to metastasis should be an important strategy for anti-metastatic treatment.

(3) **Where is the cancer cell in the way of metastasis?**

Some new methods have been found in animal experiments, and some experimental results have been achieved. However, many experimental results are difficult to pass clinical validation, because clinical validation must be observed for 3-5 years or more to evaluate long-term efficacy. Often, good results have been seen in experimental studies, but it is difficult to observe obvious effects in clinical practice. Because the laboratory subjects are animal mice, and the clinical subjects are patients, the experimental results may not be quoted in the clinic. It must be clinically proven to observe 3-5 years or even 8-10 years to understand the long-term recurrence and metastasis.

The primary or metastatic lesions of these patients have been treated properly or even satisfactorily. Why have they metastasized or even metastasized and disseminated in the future or soon? **In what form do these metastatic and recurrent cancer cells exist?** What is the cause of the transfer time of several months or years? Where are these cancer cells hidden in the human body? Why is it so stubborn? **As the common people often say: "Cancer is alive and can run." Cancer cells exist in the human body in the form of not only primary cancer and metastases, but also a third form, that is, cancer cells and cancer cell group or populations on the way.** This third form of expression has not been mentioned so far in the literature and textbooks. Because people have not yet known about it, they have neglected the special manifestation of cancer cells on the way to metastasis.

(4) **How can cancer cells survive during the metastasis?**

Although many patients use a variety of traditional treatments, radiotherapy, chemotherapy or comprehensive treatment of primary tumors or metastatic tumors, but cancer cells are still stubbornly and continuously metastasized, **then where do these cancer cells hide?** Through research, it is found that **these cancer cells can metastasize rapidly or slowly during the process of metastasis**. Under certain conditions, **sometimes they may sleep, stay in the GO phase, and sometimes the cancer cells become active and enter the cell cycle.** The "conditions" mentioned here may be related to the host's immunity, local microenvironment and other factors, and may also be related to the cell dynamics of the cancer cells themselves. **These cancer cells on the way to transfer are the most dangerous "hidden enemies".** Cancer cells that have metastatic potential during metastasis will slowly and gradually form new metastases.

The cancer cells on the way to survival can survive because it escapes the immune surveillance of immune cells in the blood circulation. If cytotoxic chemotherapy is used to treat metastatic tumors, it may be possible to further reduce the immune surveillance of immune cells in the blood circulation of patients due to the killing of excessive immune cells, and instead cause more cancer cells to escape immune surveillance during the transfer process and gradually form more new metastatic lesions.

4. the goal of cancer treatment should be directed to the above three forms of existence

Target for cancer treatment or "target or aim " of cancer treatment should be directed at three forms of cancer in the human body: one of the goals of treatment, targeting the primary lesion; the second goal of treatment is to target metastatic cancer; the third goal of treatment is to **target cancer cell populations on the way**.

(1) <u>Aiming or targeting cancer cells on the way to metastasis is just the key to anti-cancer metastasis</u>

It is proposed that the third manifestation of cancer in the human body is the multi-step, multi-factorial cancer cells, cancer cell population and micro-cancer metastasis in the process of metastasis, because this problem has not been recognized or recognized by the present. It has attracted enough attention, and there is no specific discussion on how to diagnose and treat it. In fact, the new treatment mode for coagulation, obstruction or interference of cancer cells on the way of metastasis and cutting off the metastasis pathway is the key to anti-cancer metastasis.

(2) **Aiming for cancer cells on the way to metastasis**, it may cause changes and updates in cancer diagnosis and treatment.

This new doctrine or new theoretical understanding, once confirmed by demonstration, will lead to a series of chain reaction-like cancer treatment changes and updates, such as changes and updates in the understanding of cancer treatment concepts, on cancer treatment goals or "targets" The change and update of understanding, the change and update of cancer diagnosis methods, the major changes and renewals in the research and development of anti-cancer and anti-metastatic drugs, major changes and updates on cancer treatment modes and treatment methods, As well as research on cancer metastasis and recurrence, from the cell-level pathology of cell-level oncology to molecular biology, gene expression, molecular level oncology changes and renewal.

(3) **Targeting cancer cells on the way of metastasis will bring new hope to overcome cancer**

1. Traditional cancer therapeutics believe that there are two manifestations: the first manifestation is primary cancer; the second manifestation is metastatic cancer. This traditional therapeutic concept has been in use for more than 100 years, and its therapeutic goals or "targets" target both manifestations - primary or metastatic. Treating these two "targets" in isolation does not take into account the dynamic relationship, causality, and affiliation between the two. For example, how the primary tumor is formed as a metastatic cancer, and how to stop its metastasis. Therefore, the traditional concept of cancer therapy is not comprehensive, imperfect, and defective, because it ignores cancer cells on the way to metastasis, and metastasis is the most important biological characteristics and biological behavior of malignant tumors. Without blocking the cancer cells on the way to

transfer, it is impossible to control the metastasis of cancer cells, and it is difficult to obtain the possibility of cancer treatment.

2. The new concept of cancer recognition proposed by the author is considered to have three manifestations: the first manifestation is primary cancer; the second manifestation is metastatic cancer; the third manifestation is cancer cells and cancer cells on the way to metastasis. Group and micro-cancer metastasis. This new concept is relatively complete and comprehensive. It clarifies the dynamic relationship, causality and affiliation between the three. It is a complete concept of cancer therapy, which fully explains the whole process of cancer development and how to control it. The whole process of cancer metastasis and transfer, this new theory has brought new hopes to overcome cancer.

(4) **According to the cancer cell metastasis pathway, design a new anti-metastasis treatment mode for cofferdam obstruction**

In summary, cancer treatment includes not only the surgical resection of primary tumors, surgery or radiotherapy or immunochemotherapy for the first two forms, but also the third form of treatment target or target, ie The cancer cell group on the way to transfer, carry out cofferdam obstruction, enhance the host's immune surveillance, and interfere with the prevention of cancer cell metastasis. According to the metastasis pathway of cancer cells, multi-step, multi-factor and multi-link molecular transfer mechanism of metastasis, a new anti-metastatic treatment model was designed, and new treatment methods for intervention and obstruction of cancer cells were designed.

The cancer cell group and micrometastasis on the way of metastasis have no clinical manifestations, but they do exist. Only when they enter the molecular biological level, the genetic level, or the molecular immune level can they be discovered and recognized. For example, various tumor markers that can be carried out are over-expressed. Detection of molecular immune gene changes and micrometastases. The presence of individual cancer cells (ITC) in the blood and bone marrow can be detected at the molecular level. New molecular level detection indicators, molecular immune indicators, cytokines, and tumor markers will continue to emerge. **We believe that in the near future early diagnosis of precancerous and micrometastasis will be achieved**.

8

How to stop or prevent cancer metastasis? "three steps" of anti-cancer metastasis treatment (Introduction)

1. *The steps of cancer metastasis should be understood so that it makes the cancer treatment goals more specific*
2. *Try to break each metastasis step one by one*
3. *Three major countermeasures for anti-cancer metastasis treatment ("Three Steps")*

1. The steps of cancer metastasis should be understood so that it makes the cancer treatment goals more specific

In order to make the concept of extremely complex, dynamic and continuous multi-step and multi-factor cancer cell transfer biological process clearer, the author has repeatedly considered and carefully analyzed and put forward the "eight steps" of cancer cell metastasis process. With this "eight-step" theory, the concept of understanding the complex biological processes of cancer cell metastasis is unclear and unclear. In order to carry out scientific design and intercept each transfer step, each break must have a clear and clear understanding of the concept of each step of the transfer process. Only when the "target" of each step is clear, can it be operable to study and explore. Control measures for each step.

The three-stage theory of cancer cell metastasis has been elaborated in the foregoing. One of the keys to cancer treatment is how to resist metastasis. How to carry out scientific design against metastasis is still somewhat vague and not specific enough. People only recognize the seriousness of the harm of the transfer to the patient, but lack the effective prevention and control measures with clear concept and specific structure. In order to scientifically design the interception for each transfer step. Based on this eight-step, three-stage theory and the molecular mechanism of cancer cell metastasis, the author designed and developed various stages of prevention and treatment measures, called the three-step anti-cancer metastasis treatment.

2. **try to break each metastasis step one by one**

The basic process of cancer cell metastasis is: cancer cells fall off from the primary tumor → degrade the surrounding basement membrane → migrate into capillaries, venules → surviving cancer cells adhere to capillary endothelial cells or exposed subendothelial basement membrane → through blood vessels Wall → grows in distant target organs to form metastatic cancer. This is a very complex, dynamic, continuous biological process consisting of several relatively independent and interrelated steps. In each step, a series of molecular biological events occur between cancer cells and cancer cells, between cancer cells and host cells, so that the entire metastasis process is completed and eventually metastatic cancer is formed.

In other words, cancer cells must undergo metastatic cancer at each step of the metastatic process. Failure to do so will result in the cessation of the entire transfer process. This prompts us that if we try to break each step, we will break or block the strategy of tactics for the transfer of cancer cells during the transfer process, and implement the strategy of "encirclement, chasing, blocking, and intercepting". The transfer pathway intercepts cancer cells during metastasis on the way to transfer. The new concept of cancer treatment and the new model of anti-cancer metastasis treatment are to try to block one or several steps or links of the above transfer process, so as to achieve the purpose of controlling transfer.

In order to achieve the above objectives, how should we specifically carry out anti-metastasis, what theory, what kind of technology, which drugs to use, at which step or stage and link to block cancer cells in the process of metastasis, the following will be specifically clarified.

3. **Three major countermeasures for anti-cancer metastasis treatment ("Three Steps")**

(1)   The first step of anticancer metastasis

1.   <u>The process of cancer cell metastasis at this stage:</u> cancer cells are detached from the primary tumors → adhere to the extracellular matrix (ECM) → degrade ECM, open the way for cancer cells → adhere and de-adhere through the degraded matrix, perform cell movement → then reach The outer wall of the blood vessel → degrades the basement membrane of the blood vessel → makes amoeba-like movement, first extending the pseudopod → through the blood vessel wall.

2.   <u>revention and treatment measures:</u> This stage is the intervention and suppression of cancer cells before they enter the blood vessels. The "target" of treatment during this period is mainly anti-adhesion, anti-degradation, anti-motion, anti-cancer invasion.

3.   <u>The goal of treatment is to prevent cancer cells from entering the blood vessels and achieve the goal of "being outside the country".</u>

(2) **The second step of anti-cancer transfer**

1. At this stage, the cancer cells metastasize: from the cancer cells through the blood vessel wall, into the blood circulation. Cancer cells are mixed in the blood of blood plasma and various blood cell components, or adhere to cancer cells and cancer cells to adhere to cancer cell populations, or adhere to microplates and thrombocytes, white blood cells, etc. Venous system → return to the right heart → enter the pulmonary microcirculation, some cancer cells can be parked in the pulmonary microcirculation vessels (formation of lung metastases), and some through the pulmonary microcirculation → into the pulmonary veins → back to the left heart. The cancer cells are mixed in the bloodstream through the impact of the heart valve blood flow and eddy currents, pumping into the aorta and then flowing into the small arteries of various organs → into the microcirculation of various organ tissues (especially the essential organs such as liver and kidney), brain and bone cancellous). Most of the cancer cells in the cycle are affected by immune cells or strong blood flow impact, shear damage and apoptosis. **A very small number of surviving cancer cells form tiny tumor thrombus, which can adhere to microvascular endothelial cells and degrade the basement membrane., wear out of the blood vessels**.

   At this stage, cancer cells drift in the blood circulation, contact with various immune cells, and may be captured and swallowed by various immune cells in the bloodstream to survive. A small number of surviving cancer cells escape the monitoring of immunity in the blood circulation and adhere to vascular endothelial cells.

2. Prevention and treatment measures: The "target" for treating anti-metastasis in this period is to protect and enhance the immune function of various immune cells in the blood circulation, activate immune cytokines and anti-adhesion (the cancer cells and cancer cells are homogeneously adhered, and platelets are heterogeneous Adhesion, adhesion to vascular endothelial cells) anti-motor, anti-platelet aggregation, anti-hypercoagulation, anti-cancer.

3. treatment goals: is to activate immune cells, protect the function of thymus tissue, enhance immunity, protect the marrow from blood, and promote cancer cells floating in the blood circulation for the capture, phagocytosis, encirclement and obstruction of immune cell population.

The second step is to annihilate the main battlefield of cancer cells in the blood circulation and swimming, and it is also the main countermeasure to intervene and suppress cancer metastasis.

(3)   The third step of anti-cancer transfer

1.   At this stage, the cancer cells metastasized: the cancer cells escaped the immune cell monitoring in the blood circulation and the killing of immune cells, crossed the blood vessel wall, and anchored to the local micro-environment suitable organ tissue colonization, tumor neovascularization, Metastatic metastases are formed.

2.   prevention and treatment measures: to improve the local micro-environmental tissue immunity, regulate the local micro-environment, it is not conducive to cancer cell survival implantation, inhibition of angiogenic factors, inhibition of neovascularization-based intervention, suppression measures.

In summary, the anti-cancer metastasis treatment "three-step", the space for treatment of cancer metastasis is located in the blood circulation, and the time is located at three different stages. It focuses on improving host immunity. It can be summarized as the following table and the following figure:

Table "Three Steps" for Anticancer Metastasis Treatment or Therapy of Carcinoma Metastasis

Metastasis stage of cancer cell	Metastasis process	Prevention and cure countermeasures
The stage before the cancer cell intrudes the circulation . First step of anti metastasis	Separating the cancer cell from the primary cancer→degrading ECM→adherence and de-adherence→movement→before entering the blood vessel.	• anti-adherence • anti-degradation • anti-movement • anti stroma metal protease
Transportation stage of cancer cell in blood circulation Second step of anti-metastasis	The cancer cell group and micro cancer embolus float in the blood circulation and are damaged due to being phagocytized and captured by the immunological cell and be subject to the shearing force of the blood.	• enhancing and activating various immunological cells in circulation, improving the immunologic function as the main battlefield of killing off the cancer cells in the routing of the metastasis

Authors: Xu Ze (China) ; Xu Jie(China) ; Bin Wu(America)

The stage in which Cancer cell escapes the blood circulation and anchors "target" organ
Third step of anti metastasis

After cancer cell escapes from the blood vessel, it anchors the organ for nidation, forms the new blood vessel and forms the metastatic lesion.

- anti-adherence
- anti-aggregation of blood platelet
- anti cancer embolus
- TG
- Inhibiting angiogenesis factor
- Inhibiting angiogenesis
- Improving immunological regulation
- Improving the immunity of local microenvironment.

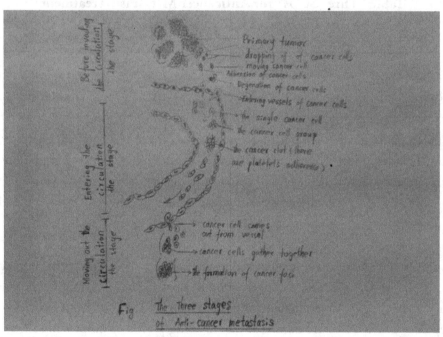

Figure Three stages of anti-cancer metastasis

(9) Cancer treatment methods and drugs (introduction)

Overview

XZ-C immunomodulatory anti-cancer traditional Chinese medicine is a traditional Chinese herbal medicine, and 48 kinds of Chinese herbal medicines with good tumor inhibition rate are screened by anti-tumor experiments in cancer-bearing mice. After compounding, the mice in the cancer-bearing mice are inhibited. In the tumor experiment, the compound tumor inhibition rate is much larger than the single drug drug inhibition rate. XZ-C1, XZ-C4 Shencao, Longyao, and Yangyangquan are composed of 28 Chinese herbal medicines, among which XZ-C1-A and XZ-C1-B100% inhibit cancer cells, 100% do not kill normal cells, and have Fuzheng This is to improve the body's immune function. From our experiments on the pharmacodynamics of XZ-C, the results of the study showed that it has a good tumor inhibition rate for Ehrlich ascites carcinoma, S180 and H22 hepatocellular carcinoma; it has obvious synergistic and attenuating effects; the experiment also proves that XZ-C immunization Regulating traditional Chinese medicine has a significant effect on improving human immune function.

After acute toxicity test in mice, there was no obvious side effects, and no obvious side effects were observed in the clinical long-term oral administration for several years (2-6 years). Simultaneous oral administration of XZ-C immunoregulatory Chinese medicine during chemotherapy can significantly reduce toxic and side effects. Oral administration of XZ-C drug during intermittent chemotherapy can increase white blood cells and increase hemoglobin. Patients with advanced cancer are mostly debilitating, fatigue, fatigue, loss of appetite, and taking XZ-C immunomodulation anti-cancer Chinese medicine for 4-8-12 weeks, can significantly improve appetite, sleep, relieve pain, and gradually restore physical strength.

It had been done the experimental research and clinical validation work.

Our laboratory conducted the following experimental studies to screen new anticancer and anti-metastatic drugs from traditional Chinese medicine:

1. In vitro screening test: In vitro culture of cancer cells was used to observe direct damage of cancer cells to cancer cells. In the test tube for culturing cancer cells, the crude drug product (500 ug/ml) was separately placed to observe whether it inhibited the cancer cells and inhibited the tumor rate.

2. in vivo anti-tumor screening test: the production of cancer-bearing animal models, the Chinese herbal medicine on the cancer screening rate of cancer-bearing animals in the experimental screening study, each batch of experiments with 240 mice, divided into 8 experimental groups, 30 per group, the first Group 7 was a blank control group, and group 8 was treated with 5-Fu or CTX as a control group. The whole group of mice were inoculated with EAC or S180 or H22 cancer cells. After inoculation for 24 hours, each rat was orally fed with crude drug powder, and the traditional Chinese medicine was screened for a long time. The survival time was observed and the tumor inhibition rate was calculated.

    In this way, we conducted a four-year experimental study. More than 1,000 tumor-bearing animal models were used each year. A total of nearly 6,000 tumor-bearing animal models were made in 4 years. After each death, liver, spleen, lung, and thymus were performed. The pathological anatomy of the kidney was performed in more than 20,000 sections.

3. Experimental results: Among the 200 kinds of Chinese herbal medicines screened by animal experiments in our laboratory, 48 kinds of positive and even excellent inhibitory effects on cancer cells were screened, and the tumor inhibition rate was above 75-90%. In this group, 152 species were eliminated from animal experiments and had no obvious anticancer effect.

| Clinical verification |

Based on the success of animal experiments, clinical validation

1. Method: Establish a combination of oncology clinic and integrated Chinese and Western medicine for anti-cancer, anti-metastasis and recurrence research, retain the outpatient medical record, establish a perfect follow-up observation system, observe the long-term efficacy, from experimental research to clinical verification, in the clinical verification process. Discover new problems and return to the laboratory for basic research, and then apply new experimental results to the clinic. Thus, the experiment - clinical - re-experiment - re-clinical. Experimental studies must be clinically validated and observed in a large number of patients for 3-5 years or even 8-10 years, according to evidence-based medicine, with long-term follow-up and evaluable data.

The standard of efficacy is: good quality of life and long survival.

RESULTS: XZ-C immunomodulatory anticancer traditional Chinese medicine preparations have achieved remarkable effects after being used in a large number of patients with advanced cancer.

2. Clinical data: Chinese and Western medicine combined with anti-cancer research collaboration group and Shuguang oncology clinic, XZ-C immunomodulation of anti-cancer Chinese medicine combined with Western medicine for treatment of stage III, IV or metastatic and recurrent cancer 4698 cases, including 3,051 males and females 1647 cases, the youngest 11 years old, the largest 86 years old, all patients were diagnosed by pathological section or CT, MRI, B-ultrasound imaging, according to the International Anti-Cancer Alliance staging criteria, all cases were intermediate stage III or higher patients, Among them, there were 1021 cases of liver cancer, 752 cases of lung cancer, 694 cases of gastric cancer, 624 cases of esophagus and cardia cancer, 328 cases of rectal cancer, 442 cases of colon cancer, 368 cases of breast cancer, 74 cases of pancreatic cancer, 30 cases of cholangiocarcinoma and 43 cases of retroperitoneal tumor. 38 cases of ovarian cancer, 9 cases of cervical cancer, 11 cases of brain tumor, 34 cases of thyroid cancer, 38 cases of nasopharyngeal carcinoma, 9 cases of melanoma, 27 cases of renal cell carcinoma, 48 cases of bladder cancer, 13 cases of leukemia, 47 cases of supraclavicular transfer For example, 35 cases of various sarcomas and 39 cases of other malignant tumors.

3. drugs and methods of administration: treatment is to protect Thymus and to increase immune function, protect the marrow from blood, thereby improving the host's immune surveillance, control the immune escape of cancer cells, from the perspective of Chinese medicine is to correct the evil, soft and loose, blood Double supplement, the drugs are XZ-C1, XZ-C2, XZ-C3, XZ-C4, XZ-C5, XZ-C6, XZ-C7, XZ-C8, ... XZ-C10,

depending on the cancer, condition, The situation of the transfer, according to the condition of dialectic, the use of the above drugs. Solid tumors or metastatic masses are all taken internally by anti-cancer powder and topical anti-cancer swelling cream. For pain, external application of anti-cancer painkiller cream, astragalus and ascites plus anti-cancer soup or water-removing soup.

4. **treatment results: improved symptoms, improved quality of life, prolonged survival.**

(1) Among the 4277 patients with advanced cancer who have been treated with XZ-C1-10 immunomodulation for more than 3 months, the medical records have detailed observation records, see the table below.

4277 cases of efficacy observation comprehensively improve
the quality of life of patients with advanced cancer

improvement	spirit	appetite	physical strength	Enhance the general situation	improve weight	Increase sleep	, improved activity, limited mobility	self-care, walking, as usual	recovery, work, light physical work
Number of cases	4071	3986	2450	479	2938	1005	1038	3220	479
(%)	95.2	93.2	57.3	11.2	68.7	23.5	24.3	75.3	11.2

This group is a middle-late stage patient, with varying degrees of symptom improvement after taking the drug, the effective rate is 93.2%. In terms of improving the quality of life (according to the Kasper's scoring standard), the average score was 50 points before the drug administration, and after the drug was increased to an average of 80 points. The patients in this group had metastasis and dysfunction of different tissues and organs in the third stage or above. It was reported that the median survival time is about 6 months. The maximum length of this group of patients has reached 18 years, and the average survival time of the remaining cases is more than 1 year. 1 case of primary hepatic lobe of hepatic lobe, recurrence of right liver after resection, treatment with XZ-C for 18 years; another case of XZ-C for 10 and a half years; 2 cases of hepatocellular carcinoma with multiple liver cancer After taking XZ-C medicine for half a year, after 2 CT examinations, the cancer lesion completely subsided and it has been stable for half a year. One case of double renal cell carcinoma, extensively transferred to the abdominal cavity after one side resection, was completely restored to work after taking XZ-C medicine. 3 cases of lung cancer open chest exploration can not be cut, long-term use of XZ-C medicine has been 3 and a half years. Two cases of residual gastric cancer were treated with XZ-C for 8 years. Three cases of rectal cancer had been treated with XZ-C for 3 years. 1 case of breast cancer metastasis of liver and ribs has been taken for 8 years. One female patient had a walnut-sized lymph node mass in both the groin and the neck. The pathological diagnosis was non-Hodgkin's lymphoma. Due to economic difficulties, chemotherapy could not be performed. Long-term service XZ-C1+XZ-C4+XZ-C2 has been 4 In the year, I went to the outpatient clinic every month to get the medicine, which is generally good. 1 case of recurrent bladder cancer after renal cell carcinoma, XZ-C drug has been used for 9 and a half years, the above cases are not surgery, can not do radiotherapy, chemotherapy, advanced patients, XZ-C drugs alone, no other drugs treatment. So far, I have come to the clinic every month to review and take medicine. After long-term medication, the condition is controlled in a stable state, so that the body and the tumor remain in a balanced state for a long time, and a better tumor-bearing survival is obtained, the patient's condition is improved, the quality of life is improved, and the survival period is prolonged.

(2) For 84 patients with solid tumors and 56 patients with metastatic supraclavicular lymphadenopathy, XZ-C series and external XZ-C3 anti-cancer light firming cream were obtained by internal administration, and the results were as follows.

Changes of 84 cases of solid tumors and 56 cases of metastatic nodules after XZ-C cream

	Solid tumor mass				supra-sacral lymph node enlargement			
	Disappear	shrink, 1/2	soft	no change	Disappear	shrink, 1/2	soft	no change
Number of cases (%)	12 14.2	28 33.3	32 38.0	12 14.2	12 21.4	22 39.2	14 25.0	8 14.2
总有效率 (%)	85.7				85.7			

298 patients with cancer pain were treated with XZ-C orally, and XZ-C anti-cancer analgesic cream was applied to achieve significant analgesic effect. See the table below.

Analgesic condition after oral administration of XZ-C and external
XZ-C anti-cancer analgesic cream in 298 patients

Clinical manifestations pain	Pain			
	Mild relief	Obvious reief	disappearance	invalid
Number of cases (%)	52 17.3	139 46.8	93 31.2	14 4.7
Total effective rate(%)	95.3%			

5. **exclusive research and development products: XZ-C immune regulation anti-cancer Chinese medicine series products (introduction)**

Authors: Xu Ze (China) ; Xu Jie(China) ; Bin Wu(America)

The self-developed XZ-C (XU ZE China) (Xu Ze-China) immunomodulatory anti-cancer series of traditional Chinese medicine preparations, from experimental research to clinical verification, applied to clinical practice on the basis of successful animal experiments, and a large number of clinical cases over the years Clinically proven, the effect is significant. For the independent invention results, it is independent innovation and independent intellectual property rights.

To search for and screen new anti-cancer and anti-metastatic drugs from traditional Chinese medicine:

The purpose is to screen out new anti-cancer, anti-metastatic, anti-recurrent and anti-cancer drugs that have no drug resistance, no toxic side effects, and high selectivity. It is well known that anti-cancer agents currently used in the world can inhibit the proliferation of cancer cells, but they kill both cancer cells and normal cells, especially bone marrow immune cells, which seriously damage the host, because the chemotherapy cell cytotoxicity is not selective. Moreover, traditional chemotherapy inhibits immune function and inhibits bone marrow hematopoietic function. Traditional intravenous chemotherapy is intermittent treatment, the interstitial period can not be treated, and the cancer cells in the interstitial period continue to proliferate and divide. Although chemotherapeutic drugs can inhibit the proliferation of cancer cells, when the cancer has not been eliminated, it has to be stopped due to its toxic side effects. After stopping the drug, the cancer cells re-growth and began to develop resistance. When resistance develops, this dose will not work, so increase the dose. However, if the dose is increased, the patient's life may be endangered. If the given chemotherapeutic drug is resistant, it will not only affect the cancer cells, but only kill the normal cells of the patient. Therefore, the cancer cells are resistant to cancer drugs and the anticancer drugs have toxic side effects on the host. It is a long-term troublesome issue. The new drug we are looking for is designed to avoid these shortcomings.

According to the theory of cell proliferation cycle, anticancer agents must be able to be used for a long time, so that the cancer can be continuously immersed in anticancer agents for a long time, so as to prevent cell division and prevent recurrence and metastasis. It must be carried out over a long period of time, and it is best to continue the long-term oral administration of drugs to control existing cancerous foci and prevent the formation of new cancer cells. However, the currently used anticancer drugs are difficult to use for a long period of time due to their large toxic and side effects, but can only be applied according to the course of treatment and short cycle. Existing anticancer drugs have immunosuppressive functions, inhibit bone marrow hematopoietic function, inhibit thymus, and inhibit toxic side effects of bone marrow. The formation and development of cancer is due to the loss of immune surveillance due to the reduced immunity of the patient. Therefore, all anticancer drugs should be to raise immunity and protect immune organs, and should not use drugs that suppress immunity.

To this end, our laboratory conducted the following experimental studies to screen new anticancer and anti-metastatic drugs from traditional Chinese medicine:

(A) Screening experimental study on the cancer suppression rate of Chinese herbal medicines by using in vitro culture of cancer cells;

In vitro screening test: The cancer cells were cultured in vitro to observe the direct damage of the drug to cancer cells.

In-vitro screening test, in the test tube for culturing cancer cells, respectively, into the crude drug product (500 ug / ml), to observe whether it has an inhibitory effect on cancer cells, we will take 200 kinds of Chinese herbal medicines that traditional Chinese medicine thinks have anti-cancer effect. Screening experiments were performed in vitro. The toxicity of the drug to the cells was tested by normal fiber cell culture under the same conditions and then compared.

(B) Making animal models of cancer-bearing animals, and conducting experimental screening of Chinese herbal medicines on the rate of tumor suppression in cancer-bearing animals

In vivo anti-cancer screening test, each batch of 240 mice, divided into 8 groups, 30 in each group, the seventh group was a blank control group, the eighth group used 5-F or CTX as a control group, the whole group of mice Inoculate EAC or S180 or H22 cancer cells. After inoculation for 24 hours, each rat was orally fed with crude drug powder, and the traditional Chinese medicine was screened for a long time. The survival time, toxicity and side effects were calculated, the survival rate was calculated, and the cancer inhibition rate was calculated.

In this way, we conducted a four-year experimental study, and conducted an experimental study on the pathogenesis, metastasis, and recurrence mechanism of tumor-bearing mice for three years, and an experimental study to explore how tumors cause host death. More than 1,000 tumor-bearing animals are used each year. In the model, nearly 6000 tumor-bearing animal models were made in 4 years. After the death of each mouse, the pathological anatomy of the liver, spleen, lung, thymus and kidney was performed. A total of 20,000 slices were taken to explore whether to find out whether There may be carcinogenic micro-pathogens, and microcirculation microscopy was used to observe the microvascular establishment and microcirculation of 100 tumor-bearing mice.

Through experimental research, we have found for the first time in China that TG has a significant effect on inhibiting tumor microvessel formation. It has been used in more than 80 clinical patients for anti-metastasis treatment, and the efficacy is being observed.

Experimental results: Among the 200 kinds of Chinese herbal medicines screened by animal experiments in our laboratory, 48 kinds of 48 kinds of Chinese herbal medicines were selected to have certain or even excellent inhibitory effects on cancer cell proliferation, and the tumor inhibition rate was above 75-90%. However, there are also some commonly used traditional Chinese medicines that are generally considered to have anti-cancer effects. After screening for animal tumors in vitro and in vivo, there is no anti-cancer effect, or the effect is very small. In this group, 152 kinds of anti-cancer effects were eliminated by animal experiments.

Authors: Xu Ze (China) ; Xu Jie(China) ; Bin Wu(America)

The 48 kinds of traditional Chinese medicines with good cancer suppression rate were selected by this experiment, and then the optimized combination was repeated to carry out the experiment of cancer suppression rate in cancer. **Finally, the immune-regulating anti-cancer Chinese medicine XU ZE China$_{1-10}$ preparation (XZ-C1-10)with its own characteristics was developed.**

XZ-C1 can significantly inhibit cancer cells, but does not affect normal cells; XZ-C4 can promote thymic hyperplasia and increase immunity; XZ-C8 can protect the marrow from hematopoiesis and protect bone marrow hematopoietic function.

Clinical validation, based on the success of animal experiments, clinical validation. That is to establish a tumor specialist clinic and a combination of Chinese and Western medicine for anti-cancer, anti-metastasis and recurrence research, retain the outpatient medical record, establish a regular follow-up observation system, and observe the long-term efficacy. From experimental research to clinical validation, new problems are discovered during the clinical validation process, and back to the laboratory for basic research, and new experimental results are applied to clinical validation. Thus, experimental-clinical-re-experiment-re-clinical, all experimental studies must be clinically verified, observed in a large number of patients for 3 to 5 years, and even clinical observations for 8 to 10 years, according to evidence-based medicine, with long-term follow-up And evaluable data, the evidence is clear that there is a good long-term efficacy, the standard of efficacy is: good quality of life, long life. XZ-C immunomodulation anticancer traditional Chinese medicine preparation has been proved to be effective after being applied in a large number of patients with advanced cancer. XZ-C immunomodulatory Chinese medicine can improve the quality of life of patients with advanced cancer, enhance immunity, increase the body's ability to fight cancer, enhance appetite, and significantly prolong survival. The introduction is as follows:

(C) XZ-C immunoregulation mechanism of anticancer traditional Chinese medicine

With the deepening of research on traditional Chinese medicine, many traditional Chinese medicines are known to regulate the production and biological activities of cytokines and other immune molecules. At this time, the immunological mechanism of XZ-C immunomodulation of anticancer Chinese medicines is elucidated at the molecular level. It is very important.

1. XZ-C anti-cancer Chinese medicine can protect immune organs and increase the weight of thymus and spleen.
2. XZ-C anticancer Chinese medicine has obvious promoting effect on bone marrow cell proliferation and hematopoietic function.
3. XZ-C anti-cancer Chinese medicine has an enhanced effect on T cell immune function, and has obvious promoting proliferation effect on T cells.
4. XZ-C anticancer Chinese medicine has a significant enhancement effect on the production of human 1L-2.

5. XZ-C anti-cancer Chinese medicine has activation and enhancement of NK cell activity, NK cells have a broad-spectrum anti-tumor effect, can kill heterogeneous tumor cells.

6. XZ-C anticancer Chinese medicine has an enhanced effect on LAK cell activity. LAK cells can kill solid tumor cells that are sensitive and insensitive to NK cells, and have a broad-spectrum anti-tumor effect.

7. XZ-C anticancer Chinese medicine has induced and induced inducing effect on interferon. IFN has broad-spectrum anti-tumor effect and immune regulation. IFN can inhibit tumor cell proliferation. IFN can activate NK cells and CTL to kill tumor cells.

8. XZ-C anti-cancer Chinese medicine promotes and enhances colony-stimulating factors. CSF not only participates in the proliferation and differentiation of hematopoietic cells, but also plays an important role in host anti-tumor immunity.

9. XZ-C anticancer Chinese medicine has the function of promoting tumor necrosis factor (TNF). TNF is a kind of cytokine which can directly cause tumor cell death. Its main biological function is to kill or inhibit tumor cells.

(D) **Biological response modifier (BRM) and BRM-like Chinese medicine and tumor treatment**

1. **Biological response modifier (BRM) has opened up a new field of tumor biotherapy. At present, BRM is widely regarded in the medical profession as the fourth program of tumor treatment.**

Oldham founded the biological response modifier (BRM) or BRM theory in 1982. On this basis, the 1984 proposed four modality of cancer treatment, biotherapy. According to the BRM theory, under normal circumstances, the dynamic balance between tumor and body defense, tumor occurrence and even invasion and metastasis are completely caused by the imbalance of this dynamic balance. If the state of the disorder has been artificially adjusted to a normal level, the growth of the tumor can be controlled and allowed to subside.

Specifically, BRM includes the following anti-tumor mechanisms:

1. to promote the enhancement of the effect of the host defense mechanism, or to reduce the immunosuppression of the tumor-bearing host, in order to achieve the immune response to cancer.

2. The natural or genetically recombinant biologically active substance is administered to enhance the defense mechanism of the host.

3. Modification of tumor cells induces a strong host response.

4. Promote the differentiation and maturation of tumor cells and normalize them.

5. to alleviate the toxic side effects of cancer chemotherapy and radiotherapy, and enhance the tolerance of the host.

2. BRM-like effect and efficacy of XZ-C immunomodulation of anti-cancer Chinese medicine

XZ-C immunomodulation anti-cancer Chinese medicine after 4 years of experimental research on cancer-bearing animals and 10 years of clinical verification showed that it has BRM-like effect and efficacy, and is a drug with BRM-like effect excavated from Chinese medicine resources. XZ-C immunomodulation anticancer Chinese medicine was experimentally screened from 200 Chinese herbal medicines by Professor Xu Ze's laboratory. Firstly, the cancer cells were cultured in vitro, and 200 kinds of Chinese herbal medicines were screened in vitro, and the direct damage of the cancer cells in the culture tube was observed, and the comparative test of the tumor inhibition rate that was measured by the chemotherapy drug CTX and the normal cells cultured as the control group was done. As a result, a batch of drugs with a certain tumor inhibition rate for cancer cell proliferation were selected. Then, the tumor-bearing animal model was further made, and the experimental study on the in vivo anti-tumor rate screening of the tumor-bearing animal model was carried out on 200 kinds of Chinese herbal medicines. The scientific, objective and rigorous experimental screening, analysis and evaluation were carried out. The results showed that only 48 species had a good tumor inhibition rate, and another 152 commonly used Chinese herbal medicines were screened by the tumor inhibition rate in this group of tumor-bearing experimental tumors, which showed no anticancer effect or a small tumor inhibition rate.

The XZ-C immunomodulatory anti-cancer metastasis drug that has been screened by the above experiments has improved immunity, increased thymus weight, protected thymus tissue function, increased cellular immunity, promoted bone marrow cell proliferation, and protected bone marrow blood production. Increase the number of red blood cells and white blood cells, enhance T cell function, activate immune cytokines, and improve immune surveillance in blood flow.

The main pharmacological action of XZ-C immunomodulation anticancer Chinese medicine is anti-cancer immune elevation, and its anti-cancer mechanism is:

1. Activate the body's immune cell system, promote the enhancement of the host defense mechanism, and achieve the immune response to cancer.
2. Activate the immune cytokine system of the body's anti-cancer mechanism, enhance the host defense mechanism and improve the immune surveillance of the immune cells of the body's blood circulation system.
3. chest lift, protect the thymus, increase immunity, protect the marrow from blood, protect the bone marrow from blood function, stimulate bone marrow hematopoietic

function, promote the recovery of bone marrow suppression, increase white blood cells, red blood cells, etc.

4. to alleviate the side effects of radiotherapy and chemotherapy, and enhance the tolerance of the host.

5. can increase the weight of the thymus, so that the thymus does not progressive atrophy, as the cancer progresses, the thymus progressively shrinks.

As mentioned above, the mechanism of action of XZ-C immunomodulatory anticancer Chinese medicine is basically similar to that of BRM, and the clinical use also obtains the same therapeutic effect of BRM. Therefore, XZ-C immunomodulation anticancer Chinese medicine has BRM-like effect and efficacy. Combining today's advanced molecular oncology theory with ancient Chinese herbal medicine resources at the molecular level, Western medicine, BRM theory as a bridge, and the international modern molecular molecular oncology advanced theory and practice.

(1) XZ-C1 "Smart Anti-Cancer"
[Main Ingredients] Eight-flavor anti-cancer medicine
[Anticancer Pharmacology]

1. Clearing away heat and detoxifying, promoting blood circulation, strengthening the body, strengthening the body, not damaging the positive, inhibiting cancer cells, inhibiting the metastasis of cancer cells, and not inhibiting normal cells.

2. The anti-cancer test in mice has inhibitory activity on mouse Ehrlich ascites cancer cells, and there is a significant difference between the drug-administered group and the control group.

3. The survival time of the cancer-bearing mice can be prolonged, and the survival rate of the mice is increased by 26.92%.

4. the main drug XZ-C1-A, XZ-C1-B has a stable and significant anti-cancer effect, 100% inhibition of cancer cells, the mitotic phase of cancer cells in the drug-administered group decreased, degeneration and necrosis were serious. It has no effect on epithelial cells or fibroblasts. Fangzhong XZ-C1-D water extract has inhibitory activity on human cervical cancer cells, and the inhibition rate of mouse sarcoma S180 is as high as 98.9%, and other flavors in the prescription also have strong anticancer effects.

5. XZ-C1 Chinese medicine on the liver cancer H22 mice anti-tumor effect: XZ-C1 medication in the second week inhibition rate of 40%, 4th week was 45%, the sixth week was 58%, the control group CTX medication The tumor inhibition rate was 45% at 2 weeks, 45% at 4 weeks, and 49% at week 6.

6. The effect of XZ-C1 Chinese medicine on the survival of H22 mice: the life extension rate of XZ-C1 group was 85%, the life extension rate of CTX control group (chemotherapy cyclophosphamide) was 9.8%, XZ-C1 treatment group

thymus Without shrinking, the thymus of the control group was significantly atrophied.

[Clinical application]

1.   **Indications: esophageal cancer, gastric cancer, colorectal cancer, lung cancer, breast cancer, liver cancer, cholangiocarcinoma, pancreatic cancer, thyroid cancer, nasopharyngeal cancer, brain tumor, kidney cancer, bladder cancer, ovarian cancer, cervical cancer, various Sarcoma and various metastatic and recurrent cancers.**

2.   **usage: XZ-C1 continuous service after 1-3 months, self-feeling effect, can be taken for a long time, after serving three years, one dose per day, after serving 5 years, can take 2 doses per week, so that immune function, cytokines long-term Maintain stability at a certain level.**

[toxicity test]

XZ-C1 can be taken for a long time. It has been shown by acute toxicity test that the mice were intragastrically administered with 104 times of adult dose (10g/Kg body weight) and observed at 24, 48, 72, 96 hours, and none of the 30 purebred mice. death. The half-lethal dose (LD50) is difficult to make and is a fairly safe prescription.

It has been used for many years in this oncology clinic. Some patients have been taking 3 to 5 years for a long time. They can also take 8 to 10 years to maintain the body's immunity and prevent recurrence and metastasis. This prescription can be taken for a long time. It is quite safe for oral cancer. medicine.

(2)   XZ-C2
[Main Ingredients] Jiuwei Anticancer Medicine
[Anticancer Pharmacology]

1.   Animal experiments can prolong the survival of L7212 mice (leukemia mice), which is statistically significant compared with the control group.
2.   can increase the inhibition rate of L7212 mice
3.   XZ-C2-A and XZ-C2-B have strong inhibitory effects on mouse sarcoma (S180).

[Clinical application]

Indications: leukemia, upper gastrointestinal malignant tumor, tongue cancer, laryngeal cancer, nasopharyngeal cancer, esophageal cancer, cervical cancer, bone metastasis.

Postoperative anastomotic recurrence and stenosis in esophageal or gastric cancer (can not be operated again).

It has a general effect on acute lymphocytic leukemia and has obvious curative effect on other types of leukemia.

Control of bone metastasis has a more significant effect.

Usage: Generally 1 capsule Qid or 2 capsules tid

Leukemia 3 capsules after tid meal, 7 days for a course of treatment.

(3) **XZ-C3 cancer pain scattered external application points**

[Main ingredients] fifteen anti-cancer drugs

[Anticancer Pharmacology]

(1) clearing away heat and detoxification, reducing inflammation and relieving pain, qi stagnation and pain relief;

(2) activating blood stasis, swelling and analgesia, a total of playing heat and detoxification, swelling and pain relief effect, and the above analgesic effect is most prominent.

(3) the application of acupoint application, than the simple application of pain, can better play the drug effect and achieve the purpose of rapid pain relief.

[Group contents] Basic side: 14 flavors such as Shannai and turmeric

[Clinical application]

Indications: liver cancer, lung cancer pain, pancreatic cancer back pain, bone cancer pain points, neck, clavicular metastatic lymph nodes.

Usage: Take a good amount of honey, mix, stir and mix into a paste. The lung cancer is applied to the root of the milk root (the 5th and 6th intercostals between the nipples), and the liver cancer is applied to the period of the door (the middle line of the milk is 6-7 intercostals).), covered with gauze after application, tape fixed, painful for 6h for 1 time, the pain is lighter, 12h replacement 1 time, continuous use until the pain is relieved or disappeared.

Experience: treatment of 84 cases of liver cancer, lung cancer pain, have analgesic effect, generally 3 times, the pain can be reduced to varying degrees, 3 to 7 days after the obvious analgesic effect, and some basic pain relief.

(4) XZ-C4 Chest Protector Free Cancer (5g/bag)

[Main Ingredients] Twelve flavors of precious Chinese herbal medicine

[Anticancer Pharmacology]

1. Promote lymphocyte transformation, enhance cellular immune function, raise white blood cells, inhibit cancer cells, and warm blood.

2. Ehrlich ascites cancer cells were transplanted into the peritoneal cavity of mice, and the mice were given chemotherapy drugs on the first day and the seventh day after transplantation. At the same time, XZ-C4 (2g/kg) was used to enhance the efficacy of chemotherapy drugs. effect.

3. chemotherapy and medicinal MMC can inhibit the leukopenia and weight loss caused by MMC.

4. Anticancer chemical drugs were injected into the veins of mice bearing cancer at the same time to take XZ-C4, and it was found that the effect of inhibiting cancer cells was more than three times higher than that of chemotherapy alone.

5. The chemotherapeutic drugs have damage to the immune organs such as thymus and spleen of the cancer-bearing mice, but after XZ-C4, the organs such as thymus and spleen do not shrink at all, indicating that XZ-C4 has a protective effect on the immune organs.

6. After giving XZ-C4 extract of Ehrlich ascites cancer mice, the life extension rate of the mice was as high as 167.1%, the survival time of the control mice was 15.2 days, and that of the XZ-C4 administration group was 25.4 days. The function of the mouse reticuloendothelial system is significantly improved.

7. XZ-C4 can make the chemotherapy drug cisplatin quickly reduce its side effects, can improve the efficacy of cisplatin. XZ-C4 can inhibit the toxic side effects of cisplatin 100%, and the dose can be a normal amount of one day. XZ-C4 does not resist the anticancer activity of cisplatin. XZ-C4 can protect the kidneys, making kidney damage of cisplatin hardly happen. XZ-C4 is a clinically promising anti-cancer disorder.

8. after the cancer surgery patients with XZ-C4 have a significant effect, after gastrointestinal, hepatopancreas and other cancer radical surgery, all showed physical decline, immunity, fatigue, fatigue, loss of appetite and anemia, etc., 1 to 2 after surgery During the week, starting from oral or gastric tube feeding, oral XZ-C4 granules, 7.5 grams per day, 3 times before meals, for 12 weeks, during which chemotherapy or immunotherapy can be performed.

9. Anti-tumor effect of XZ-C4 Chinese medicine on liver cancer H22 mice: XZ-C4 drug inhibition rate was 55% in the second week, 68% in the fourth week, and 70% in the sixth week. In the control group, the inhibition rate of CTX (cyclophosphamide) was 45% in the second week and 49% in the fourth week.

10. The effect of XZ-C4 Chinese medicine on the survival of H22 mice, the survival rate of XZ-C4 group was 200%, and the life extension rate of CTX group was 9.8%.

11. XZ-C4 can significantly improve the immune function, can increase white blood cells and red blood cells, no effect on liver and kidney function, no damage to liver and kidney sections. CTX reduces white blood cells, reduces immune function, and has kidney damage in kidney sections.

12. In the XZ-C4 treatment group, the thymus did not shrink and was slightly hypertrophied. The thymus of the control group of CTX was obviously atrophied. XZ-C4 has a strong inhibitory effect on mouse sarcoma (S180).

[Clinical application]

1. Indications: Various cancers, sarcomas, various advanced cancers, metastasis, recurrent cancer, adjuvant radiotherapy, chemotherapy, and postoperative patients. A variety of cancer can be applied, especially dizziness, fatigue, fatigue, lazy words,

less gas, spontaneous sweating, palpitations, insomnia, qi and blood are more suitable.

XZ-C4 immunomodulatory Chinese medicine, clinical and laboratory tests are performed every 4 weeks after taking the medicine and taking the medicine before surgery for 20 weeks. Check items: conscious and objective symptoms, body weight, total protein and albumin, total cholesterol, dielectric, ALT, AST blood routine and platelets, lymphocyte count, T cells and B cells, r globulin, urine protein.

Treatment results: 1 increased lymphocyte count, inhibited leukopenia; 2 has no effect on liver function; 3 has protective kidney function, does not damage the kidney; 4 can significantly reduce rash and stomatitis caused by chemotherapy and radiotherapy Etc. 5 The physical recovery of the opponent after surgery, after chemotherapy, and after radiotherapy can increase appetite, improve systemic burnout and increase body weight.

XZ-C4 is a rare and effective medicine for reducing the side effects of radiotherapy and chemotherapy and improving the overall condition of postoperative patients.

Experience: Modern medicine has proposed a variety of treatments for advanced cancer, but there are still some problems, and it is still not sure whether the combination of chemotherapy drugs for advanced cancer is effective. Even if it is effective, it also brings serious side effects. It can be considered that the treatment of cancer by modern medicine is to kill cancer cells, which is aggressive, while Chinese medicine exercises to control and even eliminate cancer by regulating the body's own regulatory functions. To this end, a treatment method that alleviates or eliminates symptoms, improves the disease or treatment, has fewer side effects, and prolongs life should be found, and XZ-C4 has such characteristics and advantages.

XZ-C4 can enhance the effect of anticancer drugs through experiments; it can promote the mitosis of B cells; it can promote the recovery of hematopoietic system of radioactive damage; promote the action of phagocytic cells; protect the thymus to raise immunity, protect bone marrow and blood The role.

[toxicity test]

XZ-C4 can be taken for a long time. Acute toxicity tests have shown that the median lethal dose (LD50) can not be done, is a safe prescription, has been used in this specialist clinic for many years, some patients take 3 to 5 years for a long time, or even take 8 to 10 years to maintain the body immunity, Prevent cancer from recurrence and metastasis. This prescription can be taken orally for a long time and is a safe anti-cancer and anti-metastatic oral medicine.

(5) The following XZ-C immunomodulatory anti-cancer traditional Chinese medicine series preparations have many experimental and clinical contents, and the length is long. Therefore, only the names are listed here, and the introduction is omitted.

1. XZ-C5 liver cancer scattered
2. XZ-C6 bladder cancer
3. XZ-C7 lung cancer scattered
4. XZ-C8 protects the marrow from blood and blood, release, chemotherapy and attenuate
5. XZ-C9 pancreatic cancer, prostate cancer
6. XZ-C10 brain tumor scattered

The above-mentioned scientific and traditional Chinese medicine preparations for anticancer, anti-metastasis and recurrence of various cancers have been applied to the oncology clinic for 20 years on the basis of experimental research, and have achieved good results.

Our traditional Chinese medicine preparation for treating various complications of cancer in our oncology clinic:

1. anti-cancer water-drinking soup - attending pleural effusion ascites
2. Shugan Jianghuang Decoction - Indications for cirrhosis and jaundice
3. postoperative cancer and health - recovery after cancer treatment
4. hunger soup - for cancer patients with loss of appetite
5. Tongyou Tang - for postoperative anastomotic stricture
6. adhesions to dissolve the soup - for postoperative cancer adhesions

The above-mentioned scientific research and test product preparations have achieved good results through the application of a large number of patients in the oncology clinic of the oncology for many years, which has alleviated the patient's pain, improved the quality of life and prolonged the survival period.

Summary table of the main pharmacological effects of Z-C immune regulation anticancer Chinese herbal medicine (anti-cancer and increasing immune)

The summary table of the main pharmacological action (anti-cancer and increasing immune function) of XZ-C immunomodulation anti-cancer Chinese herbal medicine

	Increased white blood cells	Enhanced phagocytosis	Enhance cellular immune	Enhance humoral immune	Enhanced hematopoietic function	Improve gastrointestinal function	Enhance the weight of the thymus	Promote bone marrow cell proliferation	Enhanced T cell function	Enhanced NK cell activity	Enhanced LAK cell activity	Enhanced IL-2 activity levels	Enhance the level of interferon IFN activity	Enhanced TNF activity levels	Enhanced CSF colony stimulating factor	Antagonistic WCBYC ↓	Inhibition of platelet coagulation and antithrombosis	Antitumor	Anti-metastasis	Antiviral	Anti-cirrhosis	Liver protection	Eliminate free radicals	Protein synthesis	Anti-HIV	
Z-C-A-APL																		+	+							
Z-C-B-SLT																		+	+							
Z-C-C-SNL																		+	+							
Z-C-D-PGS	+	+	+	+	+	+	6	+	+	+	+		+	+	+	+	9	+	+	+			+	+		20
Z-C-E-PCW		+	+				2	+	+			+	+	+	+	+	7	+	+	+						12
Z-C-F-AMK		+	+	+	+	+	5		+			+			+		3	+		+		+				11
Z-C-G-GUF		+	+	+		+	4			+		+				+	3	+		+		+		+		11
Z-C-H-RGL	+		+		+		3	+	+			+	+		+		5	+					+			10
Z-C-I-PLP	+	+	+	+	+	+	6		+	+						+	3	+		+					+	12
Z-C-J-ASD	+	+	+	+	+		5	+	+	+		+	+	+	+	+	8	+				+				15
Z-C-K LWF		+	+				2							+		+	2	+	+							5
Z-C-L-AMB	+	+	+	+	+		5	+	+	+	+	+	+				7	+		+				+		5

Authors: Xu Ze (China) ; Xu Jie(China) ; Bin Wu(America)

Label	1	2	3	4	5	6	N1	7	8	9	10	11	12	13	14	15	16	N2	17	18	19	20	21	22	23	24	N3
Z-C-M-LLA	+	+	+	+			4	+		+								2	+						+		5
Z-C-N-CZR		+					1					+			+			2	+	+							5
Z-C-O-PMT	+	+	+	+	+	+	6	+	+	+					+			4	+		+	+	+	+	+		16
Z-C-P-STG							0											0	+								1
Z-C-Q-LBP	+	+	+	+	+		5		+	+	+	+	+		+	+	+	8	+	+				4			16
Z-C-R-NSR		+					1	+		+						+		3	+	+		+	+				8
Z-C-S-GLK	+	+	+	+	+		5			+		+	+	+	+		+	6	+	+			+		+	+	16
Z-C-T-EDM	+	+	+	+	+		5	+		+			+	+		+	+	6	+		+			+			14
Z-C-U-PUF		+	+	+			3		+	+	+							3	+				+				8
Z-C-V-ABB							1		+	+	+			+				4	+								6
Z-C-W-SCB	+						1	+									+	2	+				+	+			5
Z-C-X-SDS							0			+	+	+						3	+								4
Z-C-Y-PAR							0			+	+	+		+	+			5	+								6
Z-C-Z-CVQ							0						+					1	+								2

76

10

Research on new concepts and new methods
of cancer metastasis treatment

A Series Products of xz-c immune regulation and control anti-cancer, anti-metastatic Chinese medication by XZ ZE exclusive research and development

Aim: To find and screen anti-cancer and anti-metastatic Chinese herbal medicines from traditional Chinese medicine

OBJECTIVE: To screen out "smart anticancer drugs" that are non-resistant, have high selectivity, are non-toxic and vice versa, and can be taken orally for a long time.

Route: From experimental research to clinical validation, the basis for success in animal experiments is applied to clinical practice

Method: To this end, we conducted an animal experiment on screening 200 new Chinese herbal medicines that traditional Chinese medicine believes have anti-cancer effects.

The author has done the following experimental research on the rate of tumor inhibition of traditional Chinese herbs

↓

(一). Cultivate cancer cells in vitro to do screen test on the rate of traditional Chinese herbs' inhibition of tumors	(二).Make the model with cancer-bearing animals inoculated with EAC or S-180 or H_{22} cancer cells to do screen test on the rate of traditional Chinese herbs' inhibiting tumors in vivo
↓	↓
Screen test on inhibiting tumors in vitro: Cultivate cancer cells in vitro and observe the direct damage of cancer cells by drugs	**Screen test on inhibition of tumor in vivo:** Make animal model, namely inoculate mice with EAC or S-180 or H_{22} caner cells
↓	↓

Authors: Xu Ze (China) ; Xu Jie(China) ; Bin Wu(America)

Screen test inside a test tube: Cultivate cancer cells inside test tubes and add crude drugs (500µg/ml); observe the inhibition of cancer cells	**Grouping:** Divide 240 mice into 8 groups in each experiment with 30 mice in a group; the 7th group is for blank control and the 8th group is used as control group with fluorouracil or cyclophosphane

Take screen tests on the 200 kinds of traditional Chinese herbs that are thought to have anti-cancer effects by traditional Chinese medicine one by one	After 24 hours from inoculation, feed the mice with specific dose of rough medical powder in a long period and observe the lifetime and untoward reactions; calculate the percentage of those whose lifetimes are prolonged and the rate of inhibiting tumors

Cultivate and test cancer cells with fibrous cell for comparison under the same condition	**Experimental results:** 48 kinds of traditional Chinese herbs do have certain rate of inhibiting tumors and 26 of them have better effects of inhibiting tumors

Experimental results: 48 kinds of traditional Chinese herbs with high rate of tumor –inhibition, other 152 kinds (that are thought to have good anti-cancer effects traditionally) have no effects on inhibiting tumors	Optimize and regroup those 48 kinds of traditional Chinese herbs with high rate of inhibiting tumors

Take a further step to make cancer-bearing animal model to do screen test on the rate of inhibiting tumors in vivo	Repeat the above experiment and the experiment on immunity

Develop Xu Ze China1~ Xu Ze China$_{10}$ pharmaceutics of traditional anti-cancer Chinese medicine for immunologic regulation and control with Chinese characteristics (XZ-C$_1$-XZ-C$_{10}$)

(五). The active principle of XZ-C traditional Chinese for immunological regulation and control can affect interleukin (IL-2)

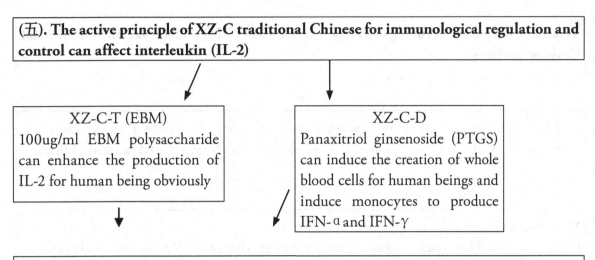

XZ-C-T (EBM)	XZ-C-D
100ug/ml EBM polysaccharide can enhance the production of IL-2 for human being obviously	Panaxitriol ginsenoside (PTGS) can induce the creation of whole blood cells for human beings and induce monocytes to produce IFN-α and IFN-γ

(六). The active principle of XZ-C traditional Chinese for immunological regulation and control can induce and promote the production of interferon.

IFN has broad-spectrum anti-tumor effects and immunological regulation; it can also inhibit the proliferation of tumor cells and activate NK cells to kill tumor cells

XZ-C-Z	XZ-C-E	XZ-C-D
250mg/kg VCQ polysaccharide can improve the level of IFN-γ produced by spleen cells.	Hydroxymethyl Poria cocos mushroom polysaccharide can regulate and control immunity, induce the production of IFN and resist virus indirectly	Panaxitriol ginsenoside (PTGS) can induce the creation of whole blood cells for human beings and induce monocytes to produce IFN-α and IFN-γ

Authors: Xu Ze (China) ; Xu Jie(China) ; Bin Wu(America)

Treatment of tumors and biological response modifier (BRM) and similar BRM traditional Chinese medicine

BRM opens up the new area of biological treatment of tumors. Currently, it has been regarded as the fourth modality of treatment of tumors which is widely appreciated in medical field.

What is BRM?
Oldham founded biological response modifier, namely theory of BRM in 1982 and proposed the fourth modality of cancer treatment, namely biological treatment later on this basis.

According to BRM theory:
Normally, tumors and the defense of organism are in dynamic equilibrium. The occurrence and even metastasis of tumors result from this dynamic equilibrium. If the disordered state can be adjusted to the normal, it is possible to control the growth of tumors and make them fade away.

The exclusively studied and developed products by the author:
according to the research on the mechanism of XZ-C traditional Chinese anti-carcinoma medicine, it is considered as that immunological regulation and control cancer invasion and metastasis are decided by the comparison of two factors, which is:
Biological characteristics of cancer cells balance leads to control
Effects of host cells by the constraints unbalance leads to the evolvement of cancer

Taked the road of modernization of traditional Chinese medicine and promoted the combination with traditional Chinese and Western medicine on the level of molecule and the connection with the modernization of international medicine.

The mechanism of XZ-C traditional Chinese anti-carcinoma medicine for immunological regulation and control is similar to that of BRM

| The effects of biological response modifier include the following:

1. To strengthen the defense mechanism of host cells or to weaken the immunodepression of cancer-bearing host cells so as to achieve immune response
2. To add natural or biological active substance with genetic recombination to strengthen the defense mechanism of host cells
3. To modify tumor cells and induce the strong response of host cells
4. To promote the proliferation and mature of tumor cells and normalize them
5. To alleviate untoward reaction of radiotherapy and chemotherapy and strengthen the resistance of host cells | The main pharmacological action of XZ-C traditional Chinese anti-carcinoma medicine is to resist cancer and strengthen immunity, whose mechanism is similar to that of BRM

1. To activate the system of immune cells and strengthen the defense mechanism of host cells to achieve the immune response to cancer cells
2. To activate the system of immune cytokine of the organismal anti-cancer mechanism to improve immune surveillance
3. To protect thymus and strengthen immunity and to protect hematopiesis of marrow
4. To alleviate the untoward reactions of radiotherapy and chemotherapy
5. To augment thymus and gain the weight to prevent its progressive atrophy and to improve immunity and immune surveillance |

As mentioned above, the mechanism of XZ-C traditional Chinese anti-carcinoma medicine is similar to that of BRM generally, which can also get analogous curative effects in clinical practice

Therefore, XZ-C traditional Chinese anti-carcinoma medicine has as analogous function and curative effects as BRM

The current molecular oncology combines with the traditional Chinese herbs to realize the combination of Chinese and Western medicine on molecular level. With BRM theory being the bridge, traditional Chinese medicine connects with international advanced theory

Authors: Xu Ze (China) ; Xu Jie(China) ; Bin Wu(America)

XZ-C$_1$ "resisting cancer intelligently"

→ **Pharmacodynamics:**
It can inhibit 96%~100% cancer cells with no effects to normal cells

→ **Pharmacology:**
It can strengthen and enhance the body resistance, and eliminate pathogenic factors without harm to body resistance. It can also inhibit cancer cells strongly with no inhibition of the normal

→ **Toxicology:**
After acute toxicity test, there is no untoward reaction. It has median lethal dose (LD50) rarely, which is a very safe drug.

XZ-C$_4$ "anti-cancer medicine for protecting thymus and improving immunity"

→ **Pharmacodynamics:**
Inhibition of H$_{22}$ mice with liver cancer:
The rate of inhibiting tumor by XZ-C$_4$ in the 2nd week is 55%
The rate of inhibiting tumor by XZ-C$_4$ in the 3rd week is 68%
The rate of inhibiting tumor by XZ-C$_4$ in the 6th week is 70%

→ **Pharmacology:**
It can promote the conversion of lymphocytes and strengthen cellular immune function. It can also increase the number of leucocytes and inhibit cancer cells so as to protect immune organs, to protect thymus from atrophy and improve immunity.

→ **Toxicology:**
XZ-C4 can be taken for a long period. According to acute toxicity test, it is difficult to get median lethal dose (LD50), so it is safe. It can be taken for 3~5 years or even 8~10 years to maintain immunity and prevent relapse and metastasis. This kind of medicine can be taken orally in a long period, which is a more effective tablet to swallow to resist cancer and metastasis.

Strive to walk the innovate road of anti-cancer metastasis with our country characters and styles

Taked the road of modernization of traditional Chinese medicine and promoted the combination with traditional Chinese and Western medicine on the level of molecule and the connection with the modernization of international medicine

The Research on New Concept and Way of Treatment of Carcinoma (6)
The Clinical Verification

XZ-C traditional Chinese medicine for immunological regulation and control has been applying to clinics after the basis of the experimental success. It has been to verify its clinical curative effects after the basis of the animal experimental success.

Building clinic for tumor speciality Building a scientific research group on anti-metastasis and relapse Building a scientific research group on anti-metastasis and relapse Building a scientific research group on anti-metastasis and relapse

↓

Keeping clinical case history Building the system of regular follow-up survey Observing the curative effects in future

↓

Keeping observing a large number of sufferers for 3~5years Or even 8~10 years clinical observation

↓

Follow-up surveys and appreciable material

↓

The standards of evaluation are good life quality and that lifetime can be prolonged

↓

After having been applied to a large number of cancer sufferers of intermediate and advanced stages for 12 years, it has achieved significant curative effects. XZ-C immunological regulation and control can be used to kill cancer cells on the way of metastasis and improve immune surveillance, which opens up the third area of anti-cancerometastasis treatment

↓

Authors: Xu Ze (China) ; Xu Jie(China) ; Bin Wu(America)

It can improve the life quality of the sufferers with intermediate and advanced stages and strengthen immunity. It can also improve the ability to regulate and control and the ability to resist cancer. By increasing appetite and physical strengthen, it can protect marrow and reinforce hematopiesis.

For those who have taken this medicine for a long period, the rates of postoperative relapse and metastasis is very low. For those who have suffered relapse and metastasis, most of them can keep stable with no further metastasis. For those who experienced several organ transplantations, it can help them stabilize the state of an illness, control metastasis and prolong lifetime.

Information of Clinical Application Verification:

Clinical information: from 1994 to Nov. 2002, XZ-C traditional Chinese medicine has been used in 4698 cases of III stage, IV stage, relapse and metastasis, in which 3051 cases are male and 1647 cases are female with the oldest being 86 years old and the youngest being 11 years old. All these have been above III stage according to TNM of International Union against Cancer by histopathology diagnosis or type-B ultrasonic, CT or MRI.

Curative effects: symptoms can be alleviated that life quality has been improved and lifetime has been prolonged. Among those 4277 cases who have taken XZ-C traditional Chinese medicine for more than three months, those with advanced cancer have had improvement of symptoms in different degree. The effective rate has researched 93.2% with general information in table 1, the improvement of life quality is seen in table 2, and the changes in tumors have been showed in table 3 and analgesia in table 4

Table 1. general information about 4277 cases of relapse and metastasis

		Liver cancer	Lung cancer	Gastric cancer	Cardia Cancer	Rectal and anal cancer	Colon cancer	Breast cancer	Cancer of pancreas
Cases		1021	752	668	624	328	442	368	74
Male: Female		4:1	4.4:1	2.25:1	3.1:1	1:1	2.1:1	All female	3.2:1
Focus	primary	694(68.8%)	699(93.9%)	-	-	-	-	-	-
	metastatic	327(31.2%)	53(6.1%)	-	-	-	-	-	-

84

General parts of metastasis		from lung (2%) from gorge (27.2%)	lymph nodes metastasis in clavicle (11.6%)	from liver (23.8%) from lung (3%)	from clavicle (13.1%)	rate of relapse (14.8%)	from liver (16.0%)	lymph nodes metastasis in clavicle (17.5%)	from liver (11.7%)
		from cardia (19.5%) from recta (31.2%)	from brain (3.1%) from marrow (4.6%)	from peritoneum(29.1%) from clavicle (6.1%)	from liver (8.3%)	from liver (7.0%)	from peritoneum (6.0%)	lymph nodes metastasis in armpit (15.0%) from bone (5.0%)	behind peritoneum (39.1%)
Age (year)	popular (%)	30-39 (76.2)	50-69 (71.6)	40-49 (73.4)	40-69 (80.4)	40-49 (75.2)	30-69 (88.0)	40-59 (65.9)	40-59 (70.0)
	youngest	11	20	17	30	27	27	29	34
	oldest	86	80	77	77	78	76	80	68

Table 2 the life qualities of the sufferers with advanced cancer among the 4277 cases with comprehensive improvement in observation of curative effects

	Spirit	Appetite	Physical strengthen	Improvement of general situation	Gain in weight	Improvement of sleep	Improvement of mobility and alleviation of movement restriction	Living by oneself and ambulating normally	Recovery of the ability to do light muscular work
Cases with improvement	4071	3986	2450	479	2938	1005	1038	3220	479
Percentage (%)	95.2	93.2	57.3	11.2	68.7	23.5	24.3	75.3	11.2

Table 3 the changes in metastatic nodes after the external application of XZ-C medicine among 56 cases

	The enlargement of lymph nodes in cervical clavicle			
	Disappear	Shrink by 1/2	Become to be soft	No changes
Cases	12	22	14	8
Percentage (%)	21.4	39.2	25.0	14.2
Total effective rate	85.7			

Table 4 the situation of analgesia after oral administration and external application of XZ-C medicine among 298 cases

Clinical performance	Analgesia			
	Alleviated lightly	Alleviated obviously	Disappear	No effects
Cases	12	22	14	8
Percentage (%)	21.4	39.2	25.0	14.2
Total effective rate	85.7			

On the aspect of improving life quality (according to KPS)

The average score is 50 before administration; it increases to 80, even 90 or 100 after 3 months

Analysis of lifetime: it is difficult to compare clinical sufferers as their stadiums and degrees are different. In this group, all sufferers are above third stage with different organ transplantations and dysfunctions. According to former statistics in this sort, the medium lifetime is about six months. In this group, the longest case is 14-years with the average lifetime of other cases being more than 1 year.

The sufferer in one case who experienced relapse and re-ablation after surgery of liver cancer has been taking XZ-C medicine for 14 years; that in another one case of liver cancer has been taking XZ-C medicine for ten and a half years; the sufferers in three cases that the lung cancer can not be cut off have been taking this medicine for three and a half years; two cases of cancer of gastric remnant taking XZ-C medicine for 8 years; three cases of rectal cancer with postoperative relapse have been taking XZ-C for 3 years; one case of mastocarcinoma with metastasis from liver and rib has been taking it for 8 years and another one case of renal carcinoma with postoperative relapse has been taking it for 9 and a half years. These sufferers have rechecked in clinic, got the medicine and taken them so as to keep the state of illness stable with lifetime being prolonged obviously.

Analysis of prolonging lifetime:

1. without surgeries, radiotherapies and chemotherapies, cases that have been taking XZ-C traditional Chinese medicine for immunological regulation and control solely for 5 years are: ① Di, central type carcinoma of lung in left top lung accompanied by metastasis in left lung, has been taking XZ-C1+XZ-C4+XZ-C7 for 5 years; ② Huang, with esophageal carcinoma has been taking this medicine for 5 years; ③ Huang with cancer in the middle place of oesophagus has been taking this medicine for 5 years; ④ Huang, with primary massive type cancer has been taking this medicine for 5 years; ⑤ Qi, primary liver cancer, has been taking this medicine for 5 years.

2. Typical cases whose cancer can not be cut off by exploratory surgeries and can not use radiotherapies and chemotherapies to treat, have been taking XZ-C traditional Chinese medicine for immunological regulation and control for 4 years: ① Cheng, with tumors after abdominal distention which can not be cut off by exploratory surgery, has been taking this medicine for 4 years; ② Fang, with cancer of pancreas which can not be cut off by exploratory surgery, has been taking XZ-C medicine for 7 years; ③ Li, with primary massive type liver cancer that can not be cut off by exploratory surgery in Tongji Hospital, has been taking XZ-C medicine for 4 years; ④ Ke, with primary liver cancer that can not be cut off by exploratory surgery in the PLA general hospital, has been taking XZ-C medicine for 5 years.

11

The formation of the theoretical system of XZ-C immune regulation and treatment of cancer

In the book "New Concepts and New Methods of Cancer Treatment", Professor Xu Ze used 30 years of self-reliance and hard work to complete the basic and clinical research of the "Eighth Five-Year Plan" of the National Science and Technology Commission. Nearly 100 research papers summarizing a series of scientific research results were published in the form of the new books.

This book has formed the theoretical system of XZ-C cancer treatment, which is the clinical basis and experimental basis for cancer treatment and has undergone the clinical application observation and verification.

XZ laboratory animal experiment found

Resection of the thymus can create a cancer-bearing animal model	As the cancer progresses, the thymus is progressively atrophied.

It was found the etiology of the cancer: **thymus atrophy, immune function is low**

It was Proposed the theoretical basis of treatment: **XZ-C immune regulation and control to protect Thymus and to enhance the immune function**

Exclusively developed products: **XZ-C 1-10 immunomodulation medications**

Clinical verification: **In the past 18 years, more than 12,000 patients with advanced cancer have been followed up in outpatient clinics, which can improve the quality of life, prolong survival and have satisfactory results.**

XZ-C theoretical system for cancer treatment
(XU ZE-China)(China-Xu Ze)

The book proposed XZ-C new concept cancer therapy, which was analyzed and compared with traditional therapy, and analyzed by table:

	XZ new concept of cancer therapy	Traditional chemotherapy and radiotherapy cancer therapy
Theoretical basis	The new concept says: Cure or Healing should be regulated and control rather than killed	The traditional concept holds or says: The goal of treatment must be to kill cancer cells
Etiology, pathogenesis	Thymus atrophy Low immune function	(——)
The theoretical basis and experimental basis of treatment	Immune regulation and control ; Protection of Thymus and Increase of immune function	(——)
Treatment principles	To Establish a comprehensive view of treatment.	Single target killing cancer cells and One-sided treatment
Treatment mode	Full treatment: surgery + biology immune regulation and control Short-course treatment: radiotherapy, chemotherapy Not long term and do not overdose	Chemotherapy + radiotherapy Or release + chemotherapy Or radiotherapy +chemotherapy synchronize
Medication therapy	XZ-C 1-10 immune regulation and control Modernization of traditional Chinese medicine and the combination of Chinese and Western medications at the molecular level	Cytotoxic drugs (both killing cancer cells and killing normal proliferating cells)

Complications, side effects	no	Toxic side effects, some have serious toxic side effects
Efficacy	Improve quality of life and prolong survival	Relieve for a few months, and may relapse
Medical expenses	Significantly reduced medical expenses	Medical expenses are large, nearly 100 billion yuan per year in China
prospect	Walked on a new way of combining immune control with Chinese and Western medicine and cancer treatment	The effect is relieved, still stagnation

II. Innovation must have challenges to traditional concepts and reform can develop

Foreword

I am a clinical surgeon. Why do you study cancer? This is due to the results of a patient interview with a group of cancer patients.

In 1985, I conducted a petition with more than 3,000 patients with postoperative chest and abdominal cancer. The results showed that most of the patients relapsed or metastasized 2-3 years after surgery, some even relapsed and metastasized several months and one year after surgery. **From the follow-up results, it was found that postoperative recurrence and metastasis were the key factors affecting the long-term efficacy of surgery.**

Therefore, we also raised an important issue: clinicians must pay attention to and study the prevention and treatment of postoperative recurrence and metastasis, in order to improve the long-term efficacy of postoperative. Therefore, it is necessary to conduct an experimental study of the clinical basis of recurrence and metastasis. Without a breakthrough in basic research, clinical efficacy is difficult to improve.

So we established the Experimental Surgery Laboratory (later established the Experimental Surgery Research Institute of Hubei College of Traditional Chinese Medicine in 1991, the research direction is to overcome cancer).

We have conducted research from the following two aspects: one is animal experimental research; the other is clinical research. Based on the success of animal experiments, it is applied clinically for clinical validation. After 28 years of hard work, a series of experimental research and clinical verification work have been carried out, and a series of scientific and technological innovations have been obtained.

Through experimental research and clinical medical practice cases, combined with the review, analysis, evaluation and self-reflection of traditional medical practice cases in the past half century, summed up the positive and negative experiences of the success and failure of clinical medical cases in the past 58 years. With the lessons, there are new discoveries, new thinking, new understandings, and new treatment concepts.

New findings in anti-cancer and anti-cancer metastasis research

First, new discoveries

A. From the results of follow-up, it was found that:

    (1)   Postoperative recurrence and metastasis are the key factors affecting the long-term efficacy of surgery.

    (2)   Clinicians must pay attention to and study the prevention and treatment measures for postoperative recurrence and metastasis.

3. From the experimental tumor research it was found:

    (1)   Our laboratory removes the thymus (Thymus, TH) from mice, and can produce a model of cancer-bearing animals. Injection of immunosuppressive agents can also contribute to the establishment of a cancer-bearing animal model. The conclusion of the study proves that the occurrence and development of cancer are obviously related to the thymus and its function of the host immune organs.

    (2)   When we explored the effect of tumor on immune organs, we found that the thymus was progressively atrophied (600 mice bearing cancer model mice) as the cancer progressed. The host thymus was acute after inoculation of cancer cells. Sexual atrophy.

    (3)   ......(6)......(omitted)

4. Through the review of clinical practice cases, analysis, evaluation and reflection of postoperative adjuvant chemotherapy cases, found that there are problems:

    (1)   Some patients with postoperative adjuvant chemotherapy failed to prevent recurrence;

    (2)   Some patients did not prevent metastasis after adjuvant chemotherapy;

    (3)   Some patients have chemotherapy that promotes immune failure.

5. Analysis from clinical practice cases, reflection on why postoperative chemotherapy failed to prevent cancer recurrence and metastasis

From the role of chemotherapeutic drugs in the cancer cell cycle to analyze, reflect; from the inhibition of the overall immune function of chemotherapeutic drugs to analyze, reflect; from the chemotherapeutic drug resistance analysis, reflection and discovery.

    (1)   There are some important misunderstandings in current chemotherapy;

    (2)   There are several major contradictions in current chemotherapy.

6. Through the review, analysis, evaluation and reflection of clinical medical practice cases, the following problems are found:

"Analysis, evaluation and questioning of systemic intravenous chemotherapy for solid tumors";

"A Century Review, Analysis and Review of the Three Major Therapies for Cancer Tradition";

"Chemotherapy needs further research and improvement."

Second, update thinking, update understanding

Through 7 years of experimental observation of cancer-bearing animals and 6 years of diagnosis and treatment of more than 6,000 cases in specialist outpatient clinics, review, analysis, evaluation and self-reflection, summarizing the experience and lessons of both positive and negative aspects of success and failure, and thinking about why traditional therapy has not significantly reduced death. Rate, why not control recurrence and metastasis? What is the problem with the traditional concept of traditional therapy. It has gradually made me realize that there may still be some problems with the current traditional cancer therapy. such as:

1. Traditional chemotherapy inhibits immune function and inhibits bone marrow hematopoietic function;
2. traditional intravenous chemotherapy for intermittent treatment, intermittent treatment can not be treated. The intermittent cancer cells continue to proliferate and divide;
3. the traditional therapy damages the host, because the chemotherapy cell poison is a "double-edged sword", which kills both cancer cells and normal cells;
4. The goal of traditional therapy is to focus on chemotherapy to kill cancer cells, but to ignore the host's own resistance to cancer, because the occurrence and development of tumors depends on the level of host immune function and the biological characteristics of the tumor itself. Both the biological characteristics of the tumor cells and the host's influence on the constraints are compared. If the two are balanced, the control is carried out, and if the two are unbalanced, the progress is made. Traditional radiotherapy and chemotherapy are all promoting the decline of immune function, which may make the two more imbalanced;
5. traditional therapy damages the central immune organs, Thymus has been inhibited in cancer, and chemotherapy inhibits the bone marrow, like "adding frost." Causing damage to the entire central immune organ without effective protection;
6. Traditional therapy is a damage therapy, which has a certain impact on the patient's disease resistance, but is not effectively protected;
7. Traditional therapy ignores the anti-cancer ability of the human body and neglects the anti-cancer system's anti-cancer system (NK cell population, K cell population, LAK cell population, macrophage cell population, TK cell population). The effects of anti-cancer cell factors IFN, IL-2, TNF, and LT in the host were ignored. Ignore the role of tumor suppressor genes and tumor suppressor gene in the host (there are oncogenes and tumor suppressor genes, cancer metastasis genes and tumor suppressor genes), neglecting the role of neurohumoral system and endocrine hormones in the host. Ignore the role of anti-cancer institutions and their influencing factors in the human body, as well as its role in regulating, balancing, and

stabilizing the host's own anti-cancer, neglecting the intrinsic factors of the body's own anti-cancer, not activated, mobilized, and only Can blindly kill cancer cells;

8. the goal of traditional therapy is relatively simple, just kill cancer cells. Not all of them meet the actual conditions of the biological characteristics of cancers that are currently recognized. Such as cancer cell invasion behavior; metastasis and multiple steps; the cause of recurrence, latent months, recurrence in several years. At present, it has been recognized that anti-tumor drugs are not necessarily resistant to metastasis, and anti-metastatic drugs are not necessarily anti-tumor.

Third, to challenge the status quo of cancer treatment, reform can develop.

How to do? Since there are problems mentioned above, further research should be carried out, basic experimental research and clinical research should be carried out, and reforms should be deepened. We should update our thinking, update our understanding, update our observations, advance in the reform, and be brave in innovation. Innovation must challenge traditional concepts, overcome its shortcomings, correct its deficiencies, and make it more perfect. Innovation must challenge the status quo and transcend the status quo. Innovation should also take a different approach and find new ways to overcome cancer.

Innovation must have challenges to traditional concepts and reform can develop

Contents

(1) Analysis, evaluation and questioning of systemic intravenous chemotherapy for solid tumors.. 101

- Analysis and questioning of the route of systemic intravenous chemotherapy for solid tumor.. 101
- Analysis and questioning on the calculation method of the dose of systemic intravenous chemotherapy for solid tumor.. 101
- Analysis and evaluation of the efficacy standard of systemic intravenous chemotherapy for solid tumors... 101

(2) Retrospect, analysis and review of the three major treatments of cancer tradition.......... 110

- Through review, analysis and reflection, discover the problems and drawbacks of traditional therapy 110

(3) Chemotherapy needs further research and improvement...124

- There are some important misunderstandings in current chemotherapy..................124
- The main contradiction of traditional chemotherapy......................................124

(4) The initiative to change the solid body tumor intravenous chemotherapy into the target organ intravascular chemotherapy 133

- Advocacy for traditional cancer therapies...133
- Assessment of problems and disadvantages of solid body tumor intravenous chemotherapy...133
- To change and perform the Intravascular chemotherapy into the target organ intravenous chemotherapy for solid tumors..133
- The initiative of specific methods and approaches of target organ intravascular chemotherapy of abdominal solid tumor 133

(5) Initiatives to strategies of improving cancer postoperative adjuvant chemotherapy.........144

- Why should cancer postoperative adjuvant chemotherapy be performed ?.................144
- The analysis of reasons why Postoperative chemotherapy did not meet the desired 144

- *how to do cancer postoperative adjuvant chemotherapy well*..................................144

(6) *The opinion of improvement and perfection of the traditional chemotherapy cancer treatment* 155

- *Discussion about the "get" and "lost" after the use of anti-cancer drugs*.................. 155
- *The status of tumor chemotherapy is the main reason for further improvement of efficacy*.. 155
- *Suggestions for improving and improving chemotherapy* 155

(7) *the basic model and specific programs of anti-cancer metastasis*..................................162

- *The basic pattern of anti-cancer metastasis* 162
- *The specific treatment plansof anti-cancer metastasis*... 162
- *Immunotherapy plays an important role in anticancer treatment* 162

(8) *the new models and new methods of cancer treatment* 168

- *Strengthen immunotherapy, to improve adverse reactions to chemotherapy*.............. 168
- *Change intermittent treatment for continuous treatment*..................................... 168
- *change the damage to the host into protecting the host*.. 168
- *change the potential of the tumor and the host, and strive imbalance into the balance* 168
- *change from damaging the central immune organs into protecting the central immune organs*.. 168
- *change the injury therapy into non-injury therapy*.. 168

(9) *"Three Steps" of Anti-cancer Metastasis Therapy*..176

- *The metastasis step should be understood so that the goal of treatment is more specific* 176
- *Try to break each step by step* 176
- *Three major strategies of anti-cancer treatment (trilogy)* 176

(10) *Review and Analysis of Clinical Cases of Adjuvant Chemotherapy for Cancer Surgery*..... 182

- *The cases of cancer postoperative adjuvant chemotherapy failed to prevent recurrence* 182

- *The cases of cancer postoperative adjuvant chemotherapy failed to prevent metastasis* 182
- *The cases of chemotherapy to promote immune failure* 182

(11)   *Review and Prospect of Treatment of Oncology Surgery* 205

- *The achievement of surgical resection of the tumor in the 20th century* 205
- *21st century surgical goal should be prevention and treatment research for cancer recurrence and metastasis after surgery radical resection* 205
- *The design of tumor radical surgery should be further studied and perfected* 205
- *The molecular biology basic research and clinical basic research of metastasis should be strengthened after the radical resection* 205
- *To prevent cancer recurrence and metastasis should be done from the surgery* 205

1

Analysis, evaluation and questioning of systemic intravenous chemotherapy for solid tumors

- *Analysis and questioning of the route of systemic intravenous chemotherapy for solid tumor*
- *Analysis and questioning on the calculation method of the dose of systemic intravenous chemotherapy for solid tumor*
- *Analysis and evaluation of the efficacy standard of systemic intravenous chemotherapy for solid tumors*

By reviewing, reflecting, summarizing, and analyzing successful experiences and failed lessons, people gradually realize that there may be some important problems in the current solid tumor systemic chemotherapy, which deserves our deep thought, evaluation and questioning.

Whether it is reasonable and scientific to use systemic intravenous chemotherapy for solid tumors, especially gastric, intestinal, hepatic, biliary, pancreatic, abdominal and other malignant tumors, should be questioned.

For the questions of the route of administration, the calculation of the dose and the evaluation criteria of the efficacy should be re-examined, analyzed, evaluated and questioned.

I. Analysis and questioning of the route of intravenous chemotherapy for solid tumors

Current status of cancer chemotherapy: mainly for systemic intravenous chemotherapy, international chemotherapy standard protocols, various joint programs or single-agent programs are also systemic intravenous chemotherapy. Systemic intravenous chemotherapy is used for leukemia, hematological malignancies, and lymphoid tumors. Solid tumors, abdominal tumors (such as stomach, intestine, liver, gallbladder, pancreatic malignant tumors) also use systemic intravenous chemotherapy. Systemic intravenous chemotherapy is also used for postoperative adjuvant chemotherapy or perioperative adjuvant chemotherapy. Is this reasonable? Is it good to learn? It should be analyzed and reflected.

(1) Analysis of the route and administration method of cytotoxic drugs for systemic intravenous chemotherapy of solid tumors

Authors: Xu Ze (China) ; Xu Jie(China) ; Bin Wu(America)

During systemic intravenous chemotherapy, intravenous infusion of drugs into the blood circulation, with the venous blood flow back to the right ventricle, and then into the pulmonary artery, after the oxygenation of the lung blood, the pulmonary veins flow into the left heart, and the heart pump is injected into the artery to enter the systemic artery. The system circulates, and the blood of the arteries of each organ is distributed to various organs and tissues of the whole body. At this time, the chemotherapeutic drug enters the extracellular tissue fluid through the capillary wall gap and then enters the cancer cell to function.

As to systemic intravenous chemotherapy, after the drug is distributed through the whole body, only a very small amount of chemotherapy cytotoxic drugs enter the extracellular tissue of the tumor, and a very small amount of drugs enter the cancer cells, resulting in minimal efficacy and effect.

Intravenous injection of chemotherapy drug via forearm vein →right ventricle →pulmonary artery→ oxygenation of pulmonary alveoli→ pulmonary vein→ aorta →systemic artery system (the drug is transported to the systemic viscera and is distributed in the whole body) →arteries of viscera→ veins of viscera →venae cavae→ right ventricle→ recirculation as above.

As above-mentioned, the drug is spread in the whole body and distributed to all viscera, in this way, the systemic viscera obtain the cytotoxic drug, however, the body surface area or volume of the solid tumor only accounts for a very little ratio of the systemic body surface area or volume, for example, even through one carcinoma of stomach as large as one adult's fist, accounts for a very little ratio of the volume of an adult. Therefore, the carcinoma of stomach as large as one adult's fist obtains a tiny minority of cytotoxic drug in the chemotherapy of systemic intravenous injection, resulting in very little curative effects or roles. Meanwhile, most of the cytotoxic drug for chemotherapy is transported to the normal histiocytes of the viscera (including heart, liver, spleen, lung, kidney, brain, bone marrow, blood, lymph and immune organ), all of which receive the cytotoxic drug for chemotherapy, resulting in side reaction. The more the times of chemotherapy, the larger the dosage, the more the drug combination, the more serious of the accumulative side reaction, even resulting in loss of immunologic function and endangering the life. The patient takes a risk of endangering the life, however, does it have curative effects on the cancerous protuberance? The carcinoma of stomach as large as a fist only can obtain a very tiny minority of dose for chemotherapy entering the cancer cells as per the body surface area, in this way, the curative effects are very little and it is impossible to realize the good curative effects.

Some patients think by mistake that the large side reaction represents the curative effects, the larger the reaction, the better the curative effects, therefore, they mistake that the reaction kills the cancer cell, but they hardly realize that the reaction kills the normal cells: it is the reaction that kills the active normal cells with normal proliferation, such as bone marrow cells, immunological cells and mucous membrane cells of the stomach and intestine and the hair, resulting in decrease of white blood cells and decrease of blood platelets. Meanwhile, no one knows whether the cancer cells are killed by the chemotherapy and how many cancer cells are killed. However, it is known that it kills the normal cells just because the decrease of white blood cells and blood platelets only indicates the completion of the chemotherapy, no one knows whether it has curative effects or not.

Therefore, we analyze the reason why the chemotherapy cannot prevent the recurrence and metastasis is possibly that the route of systemic intravenous chemotherapy does not realize the curative effects you hope and expect, the local cancer lesion is applied with a tiny minority of dose, since a very tiny minority of drug enters the external tissue fluid of the cancer cells and only a minute of dose can enter the cancer cells and takes curative effects.

An example of 5-FU, the common chemotherapy drug: 5-FU intravenous chemotherapy 1000mg/d x 5=5000mg, 85% is catabolized by DPD enzyme in the liver without any therapeutic effects; some of the rest 15% is excreted through the kidney in form of drug prototype, some enters the cells and takes curative effects through anabolism. Given the latter is 8% and the locality with easy recurrence and metastasis of carcinosis accounts for 5% of the volume of the whole body, the effective availability of 5-FU is only:

5000mg x 8% x 5%=20mg (0.4%).

In another word, when intravenous drip is used for systemic chemotherapy, chemotherapy drug 5-FU infused via intravenous drip is 5000mg, after distributed in the whole body by the viscera, the available 5-FU really reaching the cancer lesion is only 20mg, that is to say, only 0.4% of the drug reaches the cancer lesion and is utilized. The drug takes the curative effects in the cancer cells. The rest, namely 99.6% of the chemotherapy drug takes the untoward reaction in the normal cells. In other words, only 0.4% of the chemotherapy drug plays a role in killing the cancer cells while 99.6% of the chemotherapy drug kills the normal cells of the patients with active proliferation, namely bone marrow cells, epith epithelial cells of mucous membrane of the stomach and intestine, hair, white blood cells, blood platelets and immunological cells and so on, resulting in degression of immunologic function, inhibition of hematopiesis of bone marrow cells, emesis, alopecia and obvious decrease of white blood cells and blood platelets.

According to the reports of the literatures, the metabolic pathway of 5-Fu:

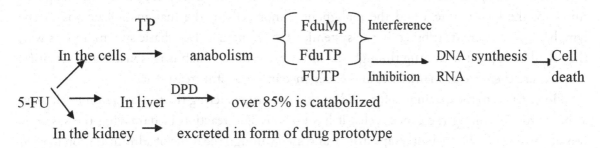

In systemic intravenous chemotherapy, how many chemotherapy drugs can reach the cancer cells and play a role in killing the cancer cells? With an example of the above-mentioned 5-FU, the patient is intravenously injected with 5000mg in 5 days, however, the one really reaching the cancer cells and playing a role is only 20mg, only accounting for 0.4% of the injected chemotherapy drug, the rest of the injected chemotherapy drug, namely 99.6% has the side effects on the normal cells with active proliferation in the whole body in clinical menifetation, namely bone marrow cells, epithelial cells of mucous membrane of the stomach and intestine and immunological cells, the systemic side reactions include arrest of bone marrow, reaction of gstrointestinal tract and toxic reaction of heart, lung and liver; the local toxic reactions include toxic reaction of skin and alopecia and so on.

In systemic intravenous chemotherapy, how does the cytotoxic drug for chemotherapy work from blood to cancer cells intravenously transfused? The chemotherapy drug is distributed and applied in the whole body, finally the chemotherapy drug enters the external tissue fluid of the cells via the interspace of capillay wall and then comes into play after entering the cancer cells.

In systemic intravenous chemotherapy, after the chemotherapy drug enters the vein, the drug is necessarily distributed in the body fluid, among the moisture in the human body, about 5% is blood, 15% is the external tissue fluid of the cells and 40% is intracellular fluid. The chemotherapy drug in blood is circulated and utilized in the whole body and distributed with the blood in the viscera. When the chemotherapy drug is in the external tissue fluid, it is absorbed and metabolized respectively by the viscera. When the chemotherapy drug enters the cells, the drug takes curative effects in the cancer cells while it takes side reaction in a large number of normal cells.

As above mentioned, we should objectively and calmly analyze the advantages, the disadvantages, the gain and the loss of the route of administration of systemic intravenous chemotherapy for the solid tumor? Which are the advantages? And the disadvantages? What the patient gains? And losses? All of which shall be seriously reflected, analyzed and evaluated.

(2) **It shall be discussed and doubted whether the route of administration of cytotoxic drug to kill the cancer cells of the solid tumor and the systemic intravenous drip are reasonable and scientific or not?**

The above-mentioned systemic intravenous chemotherapy is used for all types of leukemia, leucoma and malignant tumor in the blood system, which is reasonable just because the malignant tumor of the blood system and the malignant tumor cells of the malignant leucoma of the lymphatic system are distributed in the systemic blood system or lymphatic system, in this way, they shall be applied with drug through the intravenous drip, which is reasonable and scientific just because there are so many cases and experience in successful treatment.

However, as to the carcinoma for solid tumor, the drug entering the tumor is minute, it plays a minor role in killing the cancer cells, it has obvious side reaction in damaging the systemic proliferative cells. The chemotherapy drug transfused through the route of administration to solid tumor only can kill a tiny minority of cancer cells while most of it kills the normal proliferative cells of the host, resulting in pains from the side reaction of chemotherapy undertaken by the patients.

At present, there are so many solid malignant tumors adopting the systemic intravenous administration route for the assistant chemotherapy after operation or perioperative assistant chemotherapy. Through intravenous drip, the chemotherapy drug enters the right ventricle via the caval vein, enters the lungs via pulmonary artery, enters the left ventricle through the pulmonary vein and then is distributed in the whole body through the aorta, in this way, the chemotherapy drug reaching the cancer lesion is very little, most of the drug is distributed in the whole body and kills the normal cells, especially the immunological cells, hematopoietic cells of bone marrow, causing the patients to be severely damaged; meanwhile, it does not play a remarkable role in the solid tumor. Over half a century, it has been all the same, although it has not taken the expected effects, so many patients have suffered from the pains from the side reaction of the chemotherapy drug widely killing the normal cells. The clinicians should seriously reflect, analyze and evaluate the route of administration, which is unadvisable, unreasonable and unscientific. We shall try to apply the drug to the specific locality instead of applying drug in the whole body and we shall research it and try to correct, reform and innovate it.

II. Analysis and doubt of calculation method of the dose of systemic intravenous chemotherapy drug for solid tumor

1. Based on the above-mentioned systemic intravenous administration route, the medication is calculated as per the calculation method of leukemia, since the leukemic cells are distributed in the systemic circulatory system, the administration must cover the systemic blood system. The malignant lymphocytes of leucoma is also distributed in the systemic lymphatic system, the administration must also cover the systemic lymphatic system, the blood system and the lymphatic system are distributed in all organs, tissues and skin in the whole body, therefore the administration shall be calculated as per body surface area or volume. This kind of route of administration, calculation of dose, pharmacokinetics and bioavailability is reasonable and scientific, which conforms to the distribution of the cancer cells.

2. Since the systemic intravenous chemotherapy has taken good curative effects and experience in all types of leukemia, leucoma, epithelioma of chorion, some malignant moles, blastocytoma Wilms tumor and so on, it has been widely applied to the solid tumor of the viscera in the whole body and the assistant chemotherapy after operation, although we have accumulated much experience and obtained some achievements, we have not had our wish fulfilled just because the death rate has been not reduced, the recurrence and metastasis has been not prevented, indicating it is unreasonable to apply the calculation method to dose of the leukemia and it does not conform to the actual conditions of the solid cancer, therefore, its reasonableness and scientificalness shall be doubted and it shall be further researched for reforming and innovation.

3. Since the carcinoma of the solid tumor is restricted to the viscus before remote metastasis, it is necessary to distribute the drug to the viscus in chemotherapy, however, the drug for systemic intravenous chemotherapy is distributed in the whole body, it necessarily needs relatively more dose. However, the chemotherapy drug is the cytotoxic drug, large dose necessarily leads to large toxicity, which cannot be withstood by the patient, so the calculation of dose for systemic intravenous chemotherapy cannot be calculated as per pharmacodynamics namely how much dose is needed to kill a certain number of cancer cells, but as per the tolerance dose of the patient to the cytotoxic drug just because the patient cannot withstand it if it exceeds the tolerance dose of the cytotoxic drug as the too large toxicity will endanger the life.

Authors: Xu Ze (China) ; Xu Jie(China) ; Bin Wu(America)

In the recent 30-40 years, the systemic intravenous chemotherapy is widely used to the solid tumor or the assistant chemotherapy after operation and there have been various international chemotherapy standard schemes. the schemes and the guides indicate the kind of drug, the dose mg/m^2, from which day to which day, iv or others, indicating how many days are a cycle. The schemes are universal, no matter the side of the solid tumor, no matter whether the solid tumor is ablated or not, the schemes are all the same, the same to the calculation of the dose, which are not individualized. Since the dose determined for each scheme is determined as per the tolerance dose of the cytotoxic drug undertaken by the patient instead of the effective dose. It is calculated as per the distribution of the systemic intravenous chemotherapy in the whole body, therefore, the calculation of the dose for solid tumor and the assistant chemotherapy after operation is not reasonable and scientific just because the normal tissues of the viscera shall not be killed by the cytotoxic drug, which shall be seriously analyzed, individualized, further researched and reformed.

III. **Analysis, evaluation and doubt of curative effect evaluation criteria of systemic intravenous chemotherapy for solid tumor**

The evaluation criteria of curative effects on solid tumor at present include:

1. Size of tumor: it shall be measured in every examination.

    (1) Shrinkage of measurable volume of tumor and/or metastatic lesion: indicating the degree of shrinkage with the arithmetic product of the max. diameter (cm) and its diameter (cm) of the tumor;

    (2) As to the tumor with immeasurable size, the method for improvement of disease is the calcification of osteolytic tumor again, as to the celiac tumor that cannot be easily measures shall be expressed with the estimated shrinkage value.

2. Remission stage: the remission stage shall begin from the treatment. In both checks in the treatment stage, the tumor grows up once again, the arithmetic product of its orthogonal diameters increases over 25%. The remission stage is calculated in days, weeks or months.

3. Evaluation criteria of size of solid tumor

    CR (complete remission; evidently effective): the tumor disappears entirely, lasting over 4 weeks;

    PR (partial remission; effective): the arithmetic product of two diameters of the tumor is shrunk to over 50%;

    MR (middle remission): the tumor is shrunk to over 25% and below 50%;

NC (or S, stable, unchanged): the tumor is shrunk to below 25% and enlarged to below 25%;

PD (or P, progressive; deteriorative): the tumor is enlarged to over 25% or new lesion appears.

Analysis and discussion

1. **The above-mentioned curative effect criteria of systemic chemotherapy for solid tumor is summarized in three points: size of tumor, remission and remission period.**

Chemotherapy and radiotherapy only kill the differentiated and matured tumor cells rather than the stem cells of the tumor accounting for 0.1%~1.0% of the tumor cells. The remained stem cells of tumor are differentiated and proliferated once again, forming new tumor, with the clinical menifetation of recurrence and metastasis of tumor as well as the failure of treatment, resulting in death of the patient.

At present, although the chemotherapy drug for clinical application can shrink the tumor, the effects are commonly temporary and it cannot obviously prolong the life of the patient. Therefore, the curative effect evaluation criterion is referred to as remission, the remission stage is calculated in days, weeks or months, for example, the complete remission only means the tumor disappears entirely, lasting over 4 weeks, indicating it may recur after 4 weeks. What is meant by remission? I understand it as follows: we rope an animal, then untie it for two hours and then rope it again, in this way, the untying is referred to as remission, the two hours of untying is the remission stage, obviously, remission is not the treatment objective of the patient, the patient is hospitalized for chemotherapy, undertaking the pains and the risks from the side reaction of the cytotoxic drug for chemotherapy, only getting a temporary remission at most, which is apparentlyteh requirements and treatment objective of the patient hospitalized for chemotherapy, which shall not be the objective of clinical treatment.

2. **Why chemotherapy only can play a role in remission? Because:**

(1) The cytotoxic drug for chemotherapy only can kill the differentiated and matured cancer cells rather than the undifferentiated or immature stem cells or the ones to be differentiated and matured, the chemotherapy drug kills the differentiated and matured cancer cells at this time, however, after a time, the undifferentiated and immature cancer cells are gradually differentiated and matured, the tumor cells are uninterruptedly and progressively divided, proliferated and cloned, one is divided into two, and two into four, in this way, it is multiplied in form of geometric progression, at the same time, the period of effectively killing cancer cells of the patient through chemotherapy drug is only 1~5 days of intravenous drip, that is to say, it only lasts 5-6 days for taking the effects on killing the cancer cells, the so-called cycle of 3-4 weeks only means that the

white blood cells and the blood platelets with bone marrow inhibited can be recovered within 3-4 weeks and withstand the second chemotherapy.

(2)   Since the chemotherapy drug only can kill the differentiated and matured cancer cells rather than the undifferentiated stem cells of the tumor or the ones being differentiated, the chemotherapy only can merely alleviate the symptoms, but it cannot treat the root cause, it only can be regarded as the assistant treatment, but not as the radical treatment because the principles of chemotherapy do not conform to the biological characteristics and behaviors of the cancer cells. Although chemotherapy can temporarily shrink the tumor, it cannot obviously prolong the life and one of the reasons why the treat fails is that the tumor cells loss the drug resistance, maybe another reason is the existing therapeutic methods cannot effectively kill the stem cells of the tumor, the treatment of cancer through chemotherapy may be said that "no prairie fire can destroy the grass, it shoots up again with the spring breeze blows". Why? Because the grass is burn, but the root is remained, only some matured cancer cells rather than the stem cells of tumor to be differentiated and matured are killed, the stem cells of tumor will be continually divided and cloned in form of geometrical progression.

(3)   The judgment of the curative effects on tumor shall not regard the size of the tumor as the standard: the objective of existing tumor chemotherapy and radiotherapy is mainly to reduce the volume and number of the tumor cells just because they often determine the curative effects by means of the capability of shrinking the tumor, in fact, "the big" does not mean "the bad" and "the small" does not mean "the good". The clinic judgment of chemotherapy at present, no matter the clinic or the sickroom, is mainly based on CT and MRI as well as space occupation, as a matter of fact, the space occupation is not the size of the solid tumor because the peripheric tissue of the solid tumor may affect the space occupation. I am a surgeon and I have been engaged in medicine practice for 54 years and performed over 5000 radical and abscission operations for cancers at breast or abdomen. The size of the tumor seen in the operation has not been always consistent with the one reported in CT and MRI. In addition, although some solid tumors are as large as a fist even larger than a fist, when they are incised, the cancer cells inside is not dense while there are so many interfibrillar interstitial tissues; although some solid tumors are only as large as a table tennis, when then are incised, there are so many highly malignant cancer cells inside, the latter is more malignant than the former. Therefore, I think "the big" does not means "the bad" and "the small" does not means "the good", which cannot be regarded as the standard. We also find from a large batch of tumor-bearing animal models in the lab that although the hypodermically inoculated experimental tumors of some tumor-bearing experimental mice are very large, the cancer cells of the central tissue of the transplanted solid tumor are unlike to the peripheral cancer cells, the mode center is mostly aseptically necrotic or liquefied while its periphery is the active cancer cells, although its volume is increased, the malignancy is low.

This topic is the core content in Chapter 11 in my third book "new concepts and new methods of cancer treatment" Chapter 11 which put forward the " analysis and questioning of solid tumor systemic intravenous chemotherapy, solid tumor systemic intravenous chemotherapy drug pathways were analyzed. " Take the chemotherapy drug 5-Fu as an example:

5-Fu intravenous chemotherapy 100rng / d * 5 = 5000mg, 99.6% of the chemotherapy cytotoxic effect of intravenous drip systemic chemotherapy work on the patient's normal cells, only 0.4% of the drug to reach the foci, So its role is minimal, very little effect, too much damage to the patient. So it is put forward that : is it reasonable? Is it science?

Through this analysis and demonstration, this route of administration is unwise and unreasonable and unscientific, there is damage to the patient. Should be corrected, should be reformed, should be reformed. However, this reform will be involved in the chemotherapy in the various levels of the hospitals, involved the world's hospital oncology chemotherapy work, and should be reformed.

At present, all countries in the world, the provinces and cities around the province of the Department of Oncology and Chemotherapy are so, the solid tumor of the body intravenous chemotherapy need to get the common comments and to be a consensus, to have the gradual reform, involving very deep, very wide.

This paper is the first time in the international community that to raise this problem and the drawbacks, pointing out its shortcomings of **the use of traditional chemotherapy in the world for more than 40 years of traditional chemotherapy** - systemic intravenous chemotherapy systemic distribution, this paper is the first in the world to raise this problem, pointing out its shortcomings of the route of administration and Contradiction, that it is detrimental to the patient, and the first time in the academic community to evaluate its unreasonable, unscientific, will cause the world, the whole Chinese oncology vibration, causing tens of thousands of cancer patients shocked. (See Chapter 11, P76 in the monograph << new concept and new way of treatment of cancer>>) (here is the first published in this book **as a new doctrine for independent innovation**).

2

Retrospect, analysis and review of the three major treatments of cancer tradition

- *Through review, analysis and reflection, discover the problems and drawbacks of traditional therapy*

Three traditional cancer treatments : surgical treatment, radiotherapy and chemotherapy have been for nearly a hundred years. How are the results of these treatment? **It should conduct some centuries review and evaluation for their efficacy, from theory to practice, to the efficacy; in the future can the three major treatment be relied on to overcome cancer?how are its prospects assessed? The evaluation criteria are: reduce morbidity, reduce mortality, prolong survival, improve quality of life, reduce complications.**

We should stop and calm down and collate, analyze, review, reflect, sum up the success and failure of both positive and negative experience and lessons. What are the results? What lessons are there? Did the patient benefit? Whether is it to prolong life and reduce the pain? you should carefully analyze the successful experience, conscientiously sum up the lessons of failure, find out the problems, find out the experience and lessons. Should it think about why traditional therapy did not significantly reduce mortality? Should it think about why traditional therapy does not control recurrence and transfer? Should it think about why the three treatment has been nearly a hundred years, and now the cancer mortality rate is still the number one and the first in the city of China and township residents? I entered the Tongji Medical College for 63years and has been 60 years for cancer surgery clinical medical work and experienced and witnessed the three traditional treatments for half a century. Deeply it is thought about how to evaluate the efficacy of these treatments with the century.

What are the treatment effects of cancer patients? It is often considered to be: patients with long survival time and the good quality of life, the improved symptoms and fewer complications.

The above three traditional major means of cancer has made a brilliant contribution for the human cancer treatment,however, until the two decades of the 21st century, cancer is still rampant; the more treatment ; the more patients; the incidence of cancer continues to rise and it has high mortality and it remains the first cause of death in China's urban and rural areas.

Although the patient has undergone the regular and systemic radiotherapy and / or chemotherapy after surgery, it has not been able to prevent the recurrence of cancer cells. Why did not traditional treatment significantly reduce mortality? Does it suggest that traditional therapies do not meet the biological characteristics of cancer cells? What is the problem with traditional radiotherapy and chemotherapy? What is the traditional concept of cancer therapies? What is theoretically or conceptual problem? How can its concept or understanding of the shortcomings be corrected so that it can be the more perfect?

The review of the traditional concept

The traditional concept of cancer is the continuous division of cancer cells, proliferation; the target of treatment must be cancer cells, therefore, the traditional three treatment goals is to establish on the basis of the traditional model of killing cancer cells.

The principle basis of the current cancer is based on the following premise, that is, in order to achieve cure, it must kill the last cancer cell or the last cancer cell is killed or eliminated. Therefore, people use the expansion surgery, chemotherapy and radical radiotherapy; but the results are not ideal. In the early 1960s, the scope of tumor surgery is expanded and developed a series of radical surgery. After years of practice it is proved that to expand the scope of surgical resection, such as breast cancer, lung cancer, liver cancer, pancreatic cancer, etc failed to improve its cancer-free survival and overall survival. In the 1980s, the intensive chemotherapy and radical radiotherapy did not improve the quality of life or prolong survival, but because of severe inhibition in bone marrow hematopoietic function and immune function, it is increasing the number of life-threatening complications.

Therefore, it makes us realize that the three treatment means must be further studied and improved: the problems and drawbacks of the surgery and radiotherapy and chemotherapy should be analyzed and commented.

The reviews of surgical treatment:

Comments 1: Surgery is the effective treatment of malignant tumors, even if the cancer treatment has developed the multidisciplinary treatment today, surgery is still one of the most important and the most common means the treatment of malignant tumors and is an important part of a multi-disciplinary comprehensive treatment.

Comment 2: Surgical treatment is the main treatment of solid tumors, but the "radical surgery" design ineeds to be further studied and improved to reduce postoperative recurrence and metastasis. It should pay attention to intraoperative "tumor suppression technology" to reduce or prevent intraoperative cancer cell shedding, planting, transfer. It should pay attention to surgical operation light, stable, accurate, to reduce intraoperative promotion of cancer cell metastasis and reduce cancer cells spread from the tumor vein. To prevent postoperative recurrence and metastasis must start from surgery. It must pay attention to the non-tumor technology and to prevent the transplant and implant metastasis in the incision and drainage sites.

Authors: Xu Ze (China) ; Xu Jie(China) ; Bin Wu(America)

Comments 3: after a century of historical evaluation the solid tumor surgery is still the most important and the most reliable and it is the main treatment method which can rely on and is the main science and technology and the main treatment method for conquering cancer in the future.

Radiotherapy:

Comment 1: radiotherapy to be further studied and improved, the current radiotherapy on the patient's radiation damage protection is poor, whether for radiation diagnosis or radiation therapy, the hospital attention to the physician's protective measures, did not attach importance to the patient's protective equipment, So that patients suffer from radiation damage.

Comment 2: radiation therapy is killing cancer cells at the same time, but also killing a large number of normal tissue cells so that patients are suffering from the torture of the radiation therapy complications, the quality of life decreased, the radiotherapy and toxic effects and damage are generally persistent and irreversible, and therefore it must pay attention to the prevention of the complications of tumor radiotherapy.

Comments 3: Since the 20th century, the goal of cancer treatment is aimed at primary cancer and metastases cancer cancer cells. Despite the efforts of a century, the mortality rate of cancer still accounts for the first rate of human disease mortality, the main reason for such a high mortality rate is the transfer.

The original traditional therapy failed to reduce the long-term high mortality rate, the main reason for its failure is not for the transfer, control transfer.

Radiotherapy is the topical treatment and cancer metastasis is the systemic problems, which is a major contradiction. How to play a role in anti-metastatic therapy must be carefully considered and studied in depth.

Today, the most important problem of cancer treatment is how to resist the transfer. If you can not solve the problem of cancer metastasis, cancer treatment can not move forward. Therefore, one of the goals of cancer treatment in the 21st century should be how to prevent metastasis, but radiotherapy for local treatment, nasopharyngeal carcinoma, laryngeal cancer, lymphoma, cervical cancer, etc. have achieved good results, but it can not be anti-metastasis.

Chemotherapy:

Chemotherapy need to be further studied and improved. Does postoperative adjuvant chemotherapy prevent recurrence? Whether to prevent the transfer? How can we help prevent postoperative recurrence and metastasis, which is worthy of our in-depth thinking, research, so should come up with our own data and experience to carry out further research and refinement.

Through the review, reflection, it was summed up the analysis of successful experience and failure of the lessons, people gradually realize that in the current real truncation systemic intravenous chemotherapy there are some important problems and drawbacks worth pondering and analysis and evaluation and re-discussion.

The analysis of the problems and disadvantages of systemic intravenous chemotherapy

<u>The Analysis and evaluation and questioning of the route of systemic intravenous chemotherapy</u> for solid tumors

The current status of tumor chemotherapy is mainly systemic intravenous chemotherapy; this systemic intravenous chemotherapy route of administration is:

Chemotherapy Cell toxic drugs → Elbow Vein → Upper Venous Vein

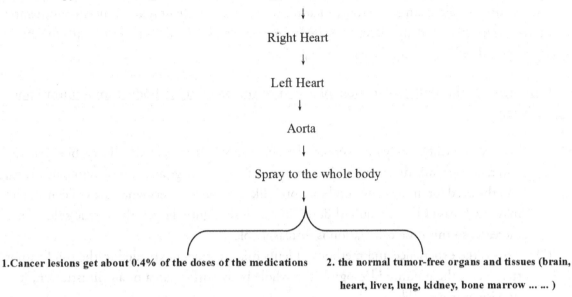

Right Heart
↓
Left Heart
↓
Aorta
↓
Spray to the whole body
↓

1.Cancer lesions get about 0.4% of the doses of the medications   2. the normal tumor-free organs and tissues (brain, heart, liver, lung, kidney, bone marrow ... ...) of the body recieved about 99.6% of the dose

Comment 1: Comment on the route of administration of systemic intravenous chemotherapy

This route of administration was not fixed-point targeted administration, but through the heart pump to the chemotherapy cell poison with the blood spray to the body so that cytotoxic has the whole systemic distribution and so that the normal organs (brain, Lung, kidney, bone marrow) of the body obtain chemotherapy cytotoxic and are damaged, leading to toxic side effects. It is very unreasonable, very unscientific, the result is:

(1) very few foci cancer can get the medications, only about 0.4%, minimal effect (due to cancer foci accounted for a very small proportion of the body surface area)

(2) 99.6% of the cytotoxic drugs are killed to the normal body of normal cells, causing brain, heart, liver, lung, kidney, bone marrow, gastrointestinal system, hematopoietic system, immune system, endocrine system toxicity.

All of these toxicity reactions are caused by the treatment design and unreasonable route of the drug administration and can be avoided.

(3) the current hospital chemotherapy drugs were not for drug sensitivity test, if the drug is resistant, then the whole chemotherapy are to kill normal tissue cells! Especially to the inhibition of bone marrow hematopoietic cells and immune cells! On the foci it is no effect! (it is in vain of that is done once a chemotherapy!)

(4)   so does every chemotherapy kill cancer cells? It does not know how much to kill? It does not know, and it can only be said to have once chemical work.

Therefore, this route of administration is unreasonable, unscientific, easily lead to iatrogenic side effects.

How to do? Should change the route of administration, to target organ tissue chemotherapy within the pathways, the drug directly to the "target organ", so the dose is very small, the effect is certain, no side effects, is conducive to the patient.

Comment 2: the dose calculation of the assessment of solid body tumor intravenous chemotherapy

(1)   because the whole body intravenous chemotherapy is not targeted delivery, but systemic coverage, systemic distribution, it is necessary to have a large amount of cytotoxic drugs, and the need for multi-drug combination is likely to make a very small area of cancer foci may reach ease Of the required dose. So the dose slightly larger, then toxic side effects increase, so this dose calculation is unreasonable.

(2)   This is the experience and methods of leukemia treatment extended to the solid tumor treatment, the guiding ideology is the whole body surface area of administration, it is unwise, unreasonable.

why?

Because leukemia cells are distributed in the systemic blood circulation system, the treatment of the "target" also exists in the systemic blood circulation system, so the use of systemic intravenous chemotherapy is reasonable, wise, but also in line with targeted therapy.

However, solid tumors are confined to an organ whose target "target" should be an organ suffering from cancer and should be targeted at the target organ's intravascular route. It should not use the leukemia treatment experience of the body surface area calculated medication, it is unwise, unreasonable.

But now solid tumors are all having systemic intravenous chemotherapy, according to the body surface area to calculate dose, in order to achieve the purpose of cancer shrinkage, the inevitable need is to increase the amount of chemotherapy cells poisoning, it will lead to more toxic side effects and complications, damage the patient.

How to do?

It should change the route of administration and change into target organ intravascular chemotherapy; this dose is very small, the effect is certain, no side effects, and is conducive to patients.

Comment 3: The Evaluation and evaluation of the evaluation criteria for the efficacy of systemic intravenous chemotherapy

The current assessment of the efficacy of solid tumors are: a, tumor size; b, remission: the general use of days, weeks, months to express.

(1)   why the evaluation of the standard as a mitigation?

At present, the clinical use of chemotherapy drugs can shrink the tumor, but the effect is usually temporary, and can not significantly extend the patient's life. Therefore, the efficacy evaluation criteria are called "mitigation". Generally with days, weeks or months to calculate, such as complete remission which is completely disappeared tumor only sustains more than 4 weeks, that is, 4 weeks later it may recur and progress.

What is mitigation? Play one by one to explain the relief, with a rope to tied up an animal, and then let it loose rope tied for 2 hours and then tied up. This release rope even if the ease of relaxation 2 hours is the remission period.

Obviously, remission is not the purpose of patient treatment; the patient is hospitalized for chemotherapy, suffering the toxicity and risk of toxic effects from chemotherapy, however it only obtains a brief remission, which is clearly not the patient to hospital treatment requirements and treatment purposes, but not the purpose of clinical care.

Mitigation, as the name suggests is palliative treatment, palliative is unable to rule, but the temporary effect, the patient to bear the pain and risk of chemotherapy cytotoxic toxicity, only for a temporary effect, ease.

(2)   why chemotherapy can only alleviate?

a.   **the effective time to kill cancer cells of the patients with chemotherapy to kill is only 3-5 days of the intravenous infusion which have the role of killing cancer cells, and then there is no the role of killing cancer cells, it is only a short time to kill about (3-5 Day), cannot once and for all, after 3-5 days the cancer cells continue to split and go on proliferation, so it can only alleviate a short time**, can not be cured, so it is ease (CR, PR) - As the name suggests, to ease is not cured and it is only the short time,that is, several weeks to get better, after this short time better, then can develop further and increase and metasatasis, therefore, to ease (CR, PR) is not the ultimate goal of treatment and not the desired purpose of the patient and the family, the patient is suffering the possible risk of the toxicity from the treatment of chemotherapy and the drug, but it only may be short-term relief. (As the following Figure 1)

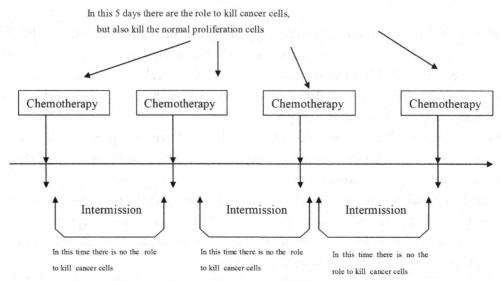

Figure 1. The action time of Chemotherapy and intermission time of Chemotherapy

So chemotherapy can not be cured and can only alleviate and can only treat the symptoms and cannot treat the reason and can only adjuvant therapy and can not cure.

So chemotherapy cannot be cured and can only alleviate and can only palliative, and can not cure and can only adjuvant therapy and can not cure.

b.   chemotherapy cell medication can only kill the differentiated mature cancer cells, can not kill yet undifferentiated and immature stem cells; this time the chemotherapy kills the differentiate mature cancer cells and after some time, those who have not yet matured stem cells gradually mature,and continue to division, proliferation, and divide into two, two for the four clones, in this way it is the geometric progression so that the foci is "wild fire burned, spring breeze and health", goes on the recurrence, metastasis and progresses. (As the following figure)

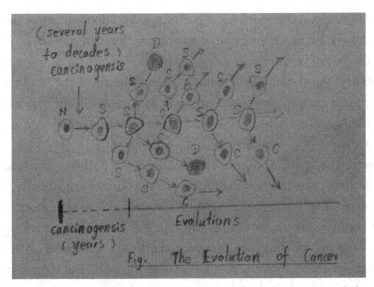

Figure 2 Cancer evolution diagram(several years to several decades)

The picture shows that the principle of chemotherapy does not meet the biological characteristics of cancer cells and biological behavior. N: Normal cells; S:stem cells; T1,2,3: mutated stem cells; 2: stem cells, 4 stem cells: polyploid stem cells; turn: the formation of metastatic cancer stem cells; R: radiation-sensitive stem cells; Resistance: drug-resistant stem cells; D: Dependent-Drug stem cells; ascites: the stem cells adapt to the growth of thousands of cells in the chest and ascites; Dead: a cell where a lethal mutation occurred ; Anti: anti-radiation of the stem cells;

Comment 4: Comment on why the adjuvant chemotherapy after the abdominal solid tumor surgery failed to prevent recurrence, metastasis?

It is because the whole body intravenous chemotherapy cytotoxic medications are injected from the superior vena cava instead of the portal vein, is difficult to reach the portal vein; the vena cava system and portal vein system are generally not connected, this route of administration is unreasonable and unscientific.

Chemotherapy is to kill cancer cells with the drugs. First of all, it must be first clear where the patient's cancer cells are in order to be targeted, clear objectives? Along the line of cancer cell metastasis line it tracks the cancer cells of being transferred in the way.

Where are the cancer cells in the abdominal solid tumor (gastric cancer, colorectal cancer, liver cancer, biliary cancer, pancreatic cancer, abdominal and other malignant tumors? It is mainly in the portal vein system, but in the current global and all of the hospital in China the abdominal solid tumor postoperative adjuvant chemotherapy is given by the elbow vein → superior vena cava → right heart → lungs → left heart → aorta → spray to the body organs. But it can not directly go into the portal vein system because the vena cava system and the portal vein system are generally not connected.

Therefore, in the abdominal malignant tumors (stomach, intestine, liver, gallbladder, pancreas, abdominal and other cancers), after the abdominal surgery the vein route of administration of the adjuvant chemotherapy injected by the elbow vein → venous is unreasonable, is unscientific, does not meet the anatomy and physiological pathology, and does not meet the reality of cancer cell metastasis pathways, because this route of administration can not directly into the presence of cancer cells in the portal vein system.

For half a century, the thousands of cancer patients in all of the world and in China are suffering from the great pain of chemotherapy cells poisoning killing the normal cells of great pain. Clinicians should seriously think, analyze, reflect and evaluate.

What should we do?

It should change the route of administration into the pathway of which chemotherapy medication is given inside the target organ vessels so that drugs can directly go into the portal vein, for the solid tumor medication should not be administered by the elbow vein, but should be changed to target organ intravascular administration, the drug targets reaching the target organ foci, which will greatly reduce the dose, improve the efficacy, will certainly reduce or eliminate the toxic side effects of chemotherapy, so that tens of thousands of cancer patients can avoid suffering from the pain and risk of the adverse reactions of chemotherapy and it is for the benefit of patients. To reduce or eliminate the toxic side effects of chemotherapy is bound to greatly reduce the medical costs and will be for the country, for patients to save more medical expenses and help solving the problem of that it is difficult to get medical treatment and the medical cost is expensive, this reform will be tens of thousands of cancer patient benefit.

Comment 5: Comment on there are some important errors in the current chemotherapy

Why did the patient postoperative chemotherapy fail to prevent the recurrence of cancer from the analysis and reflection of the clinical practice of cases?

From the analysis and reflection of the role of chemotherapy drugs in the cancer cell cycle ; from the analysis and reflection of the overall inhibition of chemotherapy to the immune function ; from the analysis and reflection of the drug resistance to chemotherapy it is found that :

(1) there are still some important errors in the current chemotherapy; the current chemotherapy still exists several major contradictions and needs to be further research and improvement.

It should be updated thinking and update awareness.

After the review, analysis, evaluation and self-reflection of 7 years of experimental experiments and 30 years of specialist outpatient clinics more than 6,000 cases of diagnosis and treatment, it is summed up the success and failure of both positive and negative experience and lessons, thinks of why the traditional therapy did not significantly reduce the death Rate? why did not it control relapse and transfer? What are the questions of the traditional concept of traditional therapy? So I gradually realize that the current cancer traditional therapies may still have some important errors. For example: ① the traditional chemotherapy suppresses the immune function and inhibit the bone marrow hematopoietic function:

It is well known that consist of central immune organs and peripheral immune organs, the former ones are thymus and marrow, the later are spleen and lymph node.

When patients are in chemotherapy, their three immune organs suffer damage (see Fig. 1), which leads to the decrease in immune function. Literature and the experimental results by the author have proved that when cancer emerges, tumors can produce a kind of immunorepressive factor (called factor of inhibiting thymus by cancer temporarily) and make thymus atrophied gradually. At the same time, chemotherapy also inhibits marrow. For the patients with cancer, the inhibition of both thymus and marrow by the chemotherapeutic cytotoxic drug make the function of the entire central immune organs inhibited, which reduces the holistic immune function as one disaster after disaster.

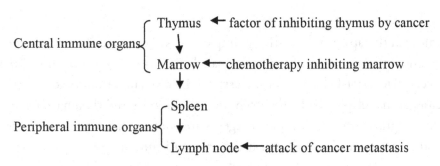

Fig 3. the damage of immune organs during chemotherapy

(2) the conventional intravenous chemotherapy is the intermittent treatment; in the intermittent period cancer can not be treated and intermittent cancer cells continue to proliferate and divide;

(3) traditional therapy damage the host, because the chemotherapy cell poison for the "double-edged sword", both kill cancer cells and kill normal cells;

(4) traditional therapy goal only focuses on that chemotherapy can kill cancer cells, while ignoring the host itself on cancer resistance and control because the occurrence and development of the tumor depends on the level of host immune function and the biological characteristics of the tumor itself, that is determined by The biological characteristics of tumor cells and the host of the constraints on the impact of the two potential, if it is the balance, cancer is controlled; if the two are imbalance, cancer is progress. Traditional radiotherapy and chemotherapy are to promote the decline in immune function and it may make the two more potential imbalance;

(5) Traditional therapy neglects the anti-cancer ability of the human body itself, ignores the role of anticancer cells (NK cell population, K cell population, LAK cell population, macrophage population, TK cell population) in the host cancer system and ignores the role of the host of the anti-cancer cytokine system IFN, IL-2, TNF, LT and ignores the role of the host of the tumor suppressor gene and tumor suppressor gene (the human body has oncogenes and tumor suppressor genes, but also cancer metastasis gene and tumor suppressor gene) and ignores the role of the neurohumoral system and endocrine hormone system in the body and ignores the role of anti-cancer agencies and their influencing factors in the human body, as well as its role of the regulation, balance and

stabilization of the host mechanism itself and ignores the inherent factors of the human body's anti-cancer activity, Blindly kill cancer cells (Figure 4)

Anticancer mechanism system → Anticancer cell system(T cell/ NK/ K /TK/LAK/Macrophage)

→ Anticancer gene system (Rb/P53/other gene)

→ Anticancer cytokine system (IFN /IL-2/TNF/LT system)

Figure 4 Schematic diagram of anti-cancer agencies

(6) traditional therapy goal is relatively simple, just kill cancer cells. And it is not consistent with the actual situation of the biological characteristics of cancer now known such as cancer cell invasion behavior; the metastasis is involved in the multiple steps; the incentives factors of the relapse can be the latent months or years and then have recurrence. It has been recognized that antineoplastic agents are not necessarily resistant to metastasis and the anti-metastatic drugs are not necessarily anti-tumor.

If there are the problems as the above-mentioned, we should further study, and we should update our thinking, update our understanding and move forward under the reform and look forward to innovate. Innovation must have the challenge to the traditional ideas and it is not substitute. But it is to overcome the shortcomings and to correct its shortcomings so that it is more perfect. Innovation also has another way and find a new way to overcome cancer. To this end, specially it is put forward the anti-cancer new ideas, new concepts, new principles, new treatment mode; according to the biological characteristics of cancer and the host's immune status and the multi-step, multi-link of metastasis it takes a comprehensive model of comprehensive treatment to be reformed, innovated and developed.

(2) to recognize that the radiotherapy and chemotherapy exist the problems and drawbacks which is difficult to be relied on conquering cancer so that it is put forward the need to launch a general attack. (Abstract, brief introduction)

(1) Review of the traditional three treatments in the century and historical evaluation

Surgical treatment:

Comment 1 - Surgery is the exact and effective way to treat cancer
Comments 2 - "radical surgery" design need to be further studied and improved
Rating 3 - Surgery is the main treatment for cancer in the future

Radiotherapy:

Comment I- does not attach importance to the patient's protective equipment and facilities

Comments 2 it must pay attention to the prevention and treatment of radiation therapy complications

Comment 3 - Radiotherapy for topical treatment, it can not be anti-metastatic, cancer metastasis for systemic problems, which is a major contradiction.

The key to cancer treatment is how to resist metastasis

Chemotherapy

Comment1: The route of administration of systemic intravenous chemotherapy is not targeted, but the whole body is distributed, and the route of administration is unreasonable, unscientific, Iatrogenic side effects. why? Because through the administration from this route 99.6% of the cytotoxic will kill normal cells, only 0.4% of the dose may kill cancer cells.

Comment 2: The evaluation of the dose of intravenous chemotherapy is to extend the experience and methods of leukemia treatment to solid tumor treatment, the guiding ideology is calculated by the body surface area, which is unwise, unreasonable, will damage Patient, easily lead to iatrogenic side effects, why? It is unreasonable because the solid tumor is confined to an organ and should not be calculated with the body surface area.

Comment 3: Evaluation of the evaluation criteria for the efficacy of systemic intravenous chemotherapy

The current solid tumor evaluation criteria are: a, tumor size; b, remission, remission (CR. PR) - As the name suggests, ease is not cured, just a few weeks of traditional put, chemotherapy goal is relatively simple, just kill cancer cells. And is not consistent with the current understanding of the biological behavior of cancer cells and biological characteristics of the actual situation.

Such as cancer cell invasion behavior; metastasis and multiple steps; relapse incentives, latent months, years and recurrence. It is now recognized that anticancer drugs are not necessarily resistant to metastasis, anti-transfer drugs do not have to kill cancer cells.

Both the above problems, should be further studied, should be updated thinking, change the concept, based on the reform, in the reform forward, innovation. Innovation, there must be a challenge to the traditional concept, to correct its shortcomings, to make it more perfect. Innovation, but also another way to find a new way to overcome cancer.

(2) to recognize the release, chemotherapy problems and drawbacks difficult to rely on the case of cancer, put forward the need to launch a general attack. (Abstract, brief introduction)

(1)　Review of the traditional three treatments in the century and historical evaluation

Surgical treatment:

Comment 1 - Surgery is the exact and effective way to treat cancer

Comments 2 - "radical surgery" design to be further studied and improved

Rating 3 - Surgery is the main treatment for cancer in the future

Authors: Xu Ze (China) ; Xu Jie(China) ; Bin Wu(America)

Radiotherapy:

Comment I- does not attach importance to the patient's protective equipment and facilities

Comments 2 1 must pay attention to the prevention and treatment of radiation therapy complications

Comment 3 - Radiotherapy for topical treatment, it can not be anti-metastatic, cancer metastasis for systemic problems, which is a major contradiction.

The key to cancer treatment is how to resist metastasis

Chemotherapy

Comment 1: The route of administration of systemic intravenous chemotherapy is not targeted, but the whole body is distributed, and the route of administration is unreasonable, unscientific, Iatrogenic side effects. why? Because of this route of administration, 99.6% of the cytotoxic to kill normal cells, only 0.4% of the dose may kill cancer cells.

Comment 2: The evaluation of the body dose of the intravenous chemotherapy of solid body tumor

The calculation of the dose is to extend the treatment of leukemia experience and methods to solid tumor treatment. Its guiding ideology is calculated by the whole body surface area. It is unwise, unreasonable, will damage the patient, easily lead to iatrogenic side effects, why? It is unreasonable because the solid tumor is confined to an organ and should not be calculated with the body surface area.

Comments 3: The evaluation of Evaluation Criteria for Evaluation of Curative Effect of Chemotherapy in the body solid tumor:

The Current solid tumor efficacy evaluation criteria are: a, tumor size; b, remission,

Relief (CR. PR) - As the name implies, the remission is not cured, Just a few short weeks of improvement. After this short-term improvement, it Will progress, increase, transfer so that the ease is not the purpose of treatment, it can not be cured and can only alleviate, and only short-term relief so that the ease is not the purpose of the patient and should not be the goal of treatment, it is unreasonable.

Comments 4

Why did the abdomen solid tumor fail to prevent recurrence, metastasis after adjuvant chemotherapy? In the Abdominal solid tumors (gastric cancer, cancer, colorectal cancer, menstrual cancer, cholangiocarcinoma, pancreatic cancer, abdominal tumor) the postoperative adjuvant chemotherapy are systemic intravenous chemotherapy, this way from the vena cava can not directly reach the portal vein. Abdominal solid tumor cancer cells mainly are in the portal vein system; the vena cava system and portal vein system is generally not connected. From the superior vena cava it is not easy to reach the portal vein so that this route of administration is unreasonable and does not meet the anatomy.

Comments 5

There are some important errors and shortcomings in current chemotherapy

a. chemotherapy inhibits the immune function and inhibits the bone marrow hematopoietic function so that the overall immune function declines, and cancer thymus is inhibited, and chemotherapy inhibit bone marrow, as "worse or snow plus frog" which all cause to damage the central immune organs and it further reduce immune surveillance; it is possible to lead that while doing chemotherapy, it has metastasis ; the more chemotherapy and the more metastasis.

b. the traditional intravenous chemotherapy is the intermittent treatment and during intermittent period cancer can not be treated, and intermittent cancer cells continue to proliferate, split, divided into two, two divided into four, cloning, and thus continue to increase the number of geometric series, Endless, spring and wind ".

c. chemotherapy only has intravenous infusion of 1-5 days, can kill cancer cells, then no killing effect, and can not once and for all, then cancer cells continue to split, proliferation, will recur, increase, so it Can only alleviate, can not be cured.

d. chemotherapy target cancer cells, is a one-sided treatment, and ignores the body's own anti-cancer ability, ignores the host anti-cancer system anti-cancer cell system (NK cells, K cells, LAK cells, macrophages), anti-cancer cells Factor gene (1FN-1L2-. ThF, LT and other factors) anti-cancer gene system (Rb gene, P53 gene), ignores the body's anti-cancer mechanism and its influencing factors, ignores the body's own anti-cancer internal factors which are not activated, mobilized, but it only blindly kills cancer cells and it is one-sided treatment view and it is very unreasonable, it does not meet the biological characteristics of cancer cells and biological behavior.

The goal of the traditional radiotherapy and chemotherapy is relatively simple and is just to kill cancer cells. And it is not consistent with the current understanding of the biological behavior of cancer cells and biological characteristics of the actual situation. For example, cancer cell invasion behavior: metastasis and multiple steps; relapse incentives, latent months, or years and recurrence. It is now recognized that anticancer drugs are not necessarily resistant to metastasis and anti-transfer drugs do not have to kill cancer cells.

Both the above problems should be further studied, should be updated thinking, change the concept, based on the reform, in the reform forward, and courage to innovation.

Innovation must be a challenge to the traditional concept, to correct its shortcomings, to make it more perfect.

Innovation should also find another way and find a new way to overcome cancer.

Such as cancer cell invasion behavior; metastasis and multiple steps; relapse incentives, latent months, years and recurrence. It is now recognized that anticancer drugs are not necessarily resistant to metastasis, anti-transfer drugs do not have to kill cancer cells.

Both the above problems, should be further studied, should be updated thinking, change the concept, based on the reform, in the reform forward, innovation. Innovation, there must be a challenge to the traditional concept, to correct its shortcomings, to make it more perfect. Innovation, but also another way to find a new way to overcome cancer.

3

Chemotherapy needs further research and improvement

- *There are some important misunderstandings in current chemotherapy*
- *The main contradiction of traditional chemotherapy*

I. Some Wrong Areas in Current Chemotherapy

1. Current chemotherapy emphasizes on only killing cancer cells and neglects to protect or even damage host cells

It is essential to attach importance to the interrelation and the interaction among host cells, tumors and drugs. Here chemotherapy is cytotoxic drug without selectivity, so it can not distinguish tumor cells and the normal with killing them together. The initial target of chemotherapy is to kill cancer cells; however, actually it also kills the proliferative cells of host cells that are damaged as a result. Especially, chemotherapy inhibits the immune system and medullary hemopoietic system of the host cells, which leads to the general decline in immune function. Consequently, that tumors are not monitored by immunity promotes the evolution of tumors. That is the reason why tumors are constringed or relieved temporary, but continue to increase and evolve after a while or even metastasize and relapse during the period of treatment. Therefore, there is one problem about chemotherapy that has not been paid much attention, namely taking no actions to protect host cells and their immune organs and immune function. The strategy of curing cancer is to destroy cancer cells protect autologous functions at the most.

2. Chemotherapy as cytotoxic drug can aggravate the inhibition on central immune organic

It is well known that consist of central immune organs and peripheral immune organs, the former ones are thymus and marrow, the later are spleen and lymph node.

When patients are in chemotherapy, their three immune organs suffer damage, which leads to the decrease in immune function. Literature and the experimental results by the author have proved that when cancer emerges, tumors can produce a kind of immunorepressive factor (called factor of inhibiting thymus by cancer temporarily) and make thymus atrophied gradually. At the same time, chemotherapy also inhibits marrow. For the patients with cancer, the inhibition of both thymus and marrow by the chemotherapeutic cytotoxic drug make the function of the entire central immune organs inhibited, which reduces the holistic immune function as one disaster after disaster.

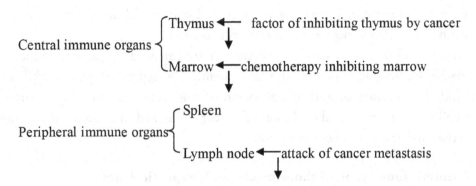

Fig. 1 the damage of immune organs during chemotherapy

Lymph nodes in peripheral immune organs as well as the areas around the focus, and lymph nodes in the process of metastasis are invaded by cancer metastasis and lost partial function, which lead to further decrease in immune function consequently. It is inevitable that tumors will evolve further, relapse and metastasize with weak immune monitor or even without it.

Due to the decline in the holistic immune function, the anti-infection ability is weakened, so chemotherapy can not continue. There may be serious complications during the process of chemotherapy, such as mycotic superinfection, viral and infectious infection. However, the antibiotics can not control them efficiently. As a result, the patients die of immune function prostration.

3. **During chemotherapy general untoward reaction may occur due to the effect of cytotoxic**

During chemotherapy, general untoward reaction can bring down immune function, and lead to arrest of bone marrow, hepatic and nephric toxic reaction, gastrointestinal response dysfunction, phalacrosis, etc. However, there is no positive and effective protection currently.

Inhibition of marrow is a usual clinic toxic reaction as marrow is the organ to store hematopoietic stem cells. It is mainly the dynamic effect of antineoplastics to the specific stem cells that chemotherapeutic drugs destroy the specific stem cells in marrow, which can reduce the number of mature and functional blood corpuscles in peripheral blood. The degree of reduction is related to the lifetime of cell components in peripheral blood, for instance, the lifetime of hematid is long, so the number of hematid in the peripheral does not change apparently; while the lifetimes of blood platelet and granular cell groups are shorter with 3 days and 67 hours respectively, so the numbers of peripheral blood platelet and granular cell groups reduce rapidly if the groups of megakaryocytic stem cells and granular cell groups are destroyed. After administering drugs, stem cells increase the time of division to make up for the amount in the process of restoration.

Authors: Xu Ze (China) ; Xu Jie(China) ; Bin Wu(America)

Most antineoplastics can result in the gastrointestinal mucosa reaction by inhibiting gastrointestinal mucosa epithelial cells.

Many kinds of antineoplastics can lead to renal toxic reaction and also affect the excretion of drugs through the kidney. It must be noticed that the damage of renal function can aggravate the general toxic symptoms or worsen the inhibition of marrow. Many kinds of antineoplastics can damage liver in different degree and affect liver function.

Such serious geneal toxic reaction of chemotherapy can lead to nausea, vomit as well as anorexia, even being unable to take food. Consequently, the general anticancer ability declines obviously and the function of anticancer system of host cells is weakened apparently. The anticancer ability of organism and evolution of cancer are locked in a "zero-sum" game, which conduce to the further development of tumors.

4. Theoretic foundation of choosing chemotherapeutic drugs

Choosing chemotherapeutic is based on cell generation cycle and pathology and physiology of cancer, or accords to the principle of pharmacokinetics. The current chemotherapeutic scheme does not always accord with the theory of cell generation cycle. During the period of treatment (3-5d), cytotoxic drugs will inhibit cancer cells. After the treatment, these cancer cells continue to proliferate and divide. Currently, the use of chemotherapeutic drugs differs in different medical institution, in which some use the treatment of 5 days, others are 3 days; some of the used drugs aim at S stage and some are for M_1 stage. No matter the treatment is 3 to 5 days or 5 days, the effective period of cytotoxic drugs on cancer cells is less than 120 hours with cell generation cycle of 50 to 80 hours, so the treatment can only act on one and a half cell generation cycles. However, the proliferating cycle of cell mass continue for years, while the effect of chemotherapeutic drugs can only last from 3 to 5 days, so the effect of killing cancer cells can just happen at the stage of proliferating cycle when the drugs take effect, such as S stage, and then disappear. After the treatment of 3 or 5 days, cancer cells continue to proliferate and divide. As a result, tumors and the metastasized lymph nodes may shrink in volume, but they are likely to augment soon.

5. Failure to take actions to control cancer cells continuously and consolidate the effect at the interval of two times of chemotherapies

The treatment between two times of chemotherapies is blank, and the actions to continuous killing or control on cancer cells are not taken to consolidate the curative effect. What have been done is waiting the restoration of leucocytes and blood platelets to achieve the aim of stand chemotherapy next time. Actually, the treatment at the interval is very important, for cancer cells are out of control and proliferate and divide further positively and potentially at intervals due to the heavy decline in immune function. The more times of chemotherapies and the larger dosage of drugs, the more cytotoxic drugs will be used correspondently, so that the general immune function is worse and worse and the immunity of organism is less and less able to control the proliferation of oncocytes and prevent the metastasis leading to relapse and metastasize after continuous chemotherapies. Therefore, it is necessary to adopt immunological therapy or Chinese traditional medicine for regulating immunity to avoid relapse.

6. **Theoretical foundation of postoperative auxiliary chemotherapy, the length of the intervals between two times of chemotherapies and the time of chemotherapy**

The arrangements of chemotherapy differ in different locations and medical institutions, among which some use once a month or once every two months, some adopt six times in a row, or continuous four or eight times. The treatment is much blinder, especially postoperative auxiliary chemotherapy. The current arrangement of chemotherapeutic period is that only when leucocyte and blood platelet restore, can the next chemotherapy be taken. In fact, it is more helpless instead of meeting the pathological and physical demands (since the time of restoration is longer for some patients, when cancer cells have been in the process of division and proliferation continuously). What is the aim of auxiliary chemotherapy? How to achieve the aim? Are there any residual cancer cells in the body although the aim of chemotherapy is to kill cancer cells? Where do the cancer cells hide after surgeons, in the local of the surgeon, lymph nodes or in the blood? Taking gastrointestinal surgeon for instance, do the residual cancer cells hide in portal vein blood, or in celiac lymph nodes, or even in the local area of the surgeon? How long can the residual cancer cells lurk after surgeons before devastated by host cells? How to arrange the period of postoperative auxiliary chemotherapy? Knowing the location of cancer cells may be good for controlling the residual cancer cells in the area of surgeons and portal vein.

In a word, the current choice of postoperative auxiliary chemotherapy and the arrangement of chemotherapeutic period are very blind. It is essential to do further clinic research to ensure the indication, contraindication, medication and route of administration as well as a more uniform scheme so as to conclude analysis and evaluate.

7. **Blindness of current chemotherapy**

It may be helpful for some patients to take on chemotherapy blindly just according to experience, but it is harmful for a considerable number of patients. For instance, if some patient was resistant to this kind of drug, it would be harmful, rather than fruitless, for the cytotoxic drugs of chemotherapy can not act on cancer cells, instead of killing normal histiocyte, especially immunocyte, myeloid cell, which will lead to the prostration of immune function.

Drugsensitive test is a must to verify whether the patient is allergic to the used drugs. Only doing like this can ensure the accuracy of administering drugs. Currently, it is common that clinical administrate of drugs depends on experience blindly. Such blind administrate is potentially dangerous. If the drug is really sensitive to the patient's cancer cells, it will be effective (CR, PR). But if the drug is not sensitive to the cancer cells, it will only kill the normal cells and inhibit the marrow hematopiesis leading to the reduction in leucocyte and blood platelet as well as the decline in immune function without any damage on cancer cells, which will definitely promote the evolution of tumors and result in the prostration of immune function and hematopiesis. The decrease in immune function makes tumors be beyond the immune monitor and develop further, and then promote the relapse and metastasis. Therefore, it is necessary to take on individual drugsensitive test and drug resistant test.

8. Cure of cancer aims to kill tumors, reserve organism and regain health

The cure of cancer should always run through both strengthening health and wiping evil off, in which wiping evil off means inhibiting and killing cancer cells, clearing up lumps; strengthening health means protecting organismal ability to recognize dissidents, exciting the organismal positive factors of anti-cancer and improve the organismal ability to resist cancer. These two are dialectic and united. However, the current treatment on cancer only emphasizes killing cancer cells and ignores the protection of host cells, which damages the immune system and the system of marrow hematopiesis resulting in wiping both evil and health away. If tumors are drug resistant to this chemotherapeutic drug, it is likely to be harmful to health without wiping evil away. The treatment on cancer needs a scientific designed scheme, for cancer results from losing the balance between the organismal immune capacity of anti-cancer and the development of tumors, and from losing immune monitor, which leads to the further development of tumors. So it is necessary to try to restore the balance. Taking teeterboard in a children's playground for instance, tumor and the immunity of host cells represent the two ends of a teeterboard respectively. The comparison of the two parties' power decides the direction of tilt and the final result. Besides, the example of "scale" can be explained in the same way. However, chemotherapy does not emphasize the protection of host cells but promotes the diffuse and evolution of tumors.

9. Standards for the curative effects of chemotherapy should be good quality of life and prolonged lifetime

How to evaluate the curative effect of postoperative auxiliary chemotherapy? As the tumor has been ablated, it is unable to evaluate the effect in terms of its shrink.

Most patients only regard untoward reactions after chemotherapy, like decline in leucocyte and blood platelet, nausea and disgorge, anorexia, hypodynamia and abdominal distention as the curative effects, but they hardly realize that these symptoms are not the effects at all. It is unable to evaluate the postoperative curative effects until now. The current diagnostic methods are still laggard, as when tumors are detected, they have been very serious. Therefore, molecular biology is the only way to solve this problem.

Generally speaking, the standard for curative effects is remission. In terms of remission, the efficiency is defined as the shrink of the tumor, however, the quality of life is not improved and the lifetime is not prolonged, which is not the aim of handling diseases for the patients with cancer.

10. **Anti-Carcinomatous drugs used currently can not always resist metastasis and relapse and the drugs for anti- carcinomatous metastasis and anti-cancer should be different**

For many cases, postoperative auxiliary can not prevent relapse and metastasis, which relates to the fact that the current anti- carcinomatous drugs are not always able to resist metastasis and relapse besides other various possible factors mentioned above. Drugs for anti-metastasis should be different from anti-carcinomatous drugs as generally anti-cancer drugs have cytotoxicity and aim at killing cancer cells, destroying and inhibiting cell division and proliferation, whereas drugs for resisting metastasis are mainly used to resist the invasion of tumor cells, to antagonize the adherence of cancer cells inside the blood vessels, to inhibit the nascent micrangium and strengthen the organismal immunity to kill cancer cells. Most of anti- carcinomatous metastasis drugs have no cytotoxicity.

Research on anti-cancer drugs has stepped into a new stage. It is confronted with theoretical and technical renovations and the change in the train of thoughts when the field of research on anti-cancer drugs is not restricted to the traditional thoughts based on cytotoxic and the working method of cytotoxic drugs. New methods like inducement of differentiate, regulator of biological reaction, immunoregulation, genetherapy, combination of Chinese and western medicine, etc. have been taken into consideration in succession.

Although chemotherapy has been applied for sixty years, it is not satisfactory that many problems still exist reflected by the statistic, analysis and evaluation of applied information from a large number of clinical suffers. It is pitiful that cancer may metastasize and relapse after or during the process of chemotherapy.

In conclusion, the possible reasons that postoperative auxiliary chemotherapy is unable to prevent relapse and metastasis are, ①chemotherapeutant can promote the decline in immune function and inhibit hematopoiesis of marrow; ②failure to continue aftertreatment at the intervals of chemotherapies; ③chemotherapeutic drugs can not protect host cells; ④lumps may has drug resistance; ⑤chemotherapeutic drugs may be not sensitive; ⑥chemotherapeutic drugs for solid tumor may be not infiltrate into tumors; ⑦the arrangement of chemotherapeutic period is not reasonable; ⑧drugs may not act on the sensitive period of cell proliferation; ⑨it is difficult to restore immune function and hematopoiesis probably.

II. The Main Contradictions in Traditional Chemotherapy

So far, the aim of chemotherapy has been still focusing on killing cancer cells. The majority of chemotherapeutic drugs are cytotoxic drugs without selectivity, so both cancer cells and normal ones will be damaged. Besides, chemotherapy has serious untoward reaction, suffers will have intensive feeling and have to give up the treatment at last. In the last ten years, the author has helped nearly ten thousand cancer cases in Wuchang Shuguang Tumorous Clinic, many of whom have tried chemotherapy. They came to anti-carcinomatous clinic for treatment as there were no curative effects after several periods of treatment. It can be implicated that auxiliary treatment does not prevent carcinomatous invasion, relapse and metastasis, and it also can not improve the quality of life and prolong lifetime obviously. Through the feedback of those cases, analysis, evaluation and reflection, the author have recognized that there are the following contradictions in traditional chemotherapy.

1. The contradiction between chemotherapeutic cytotoxic and the damage to host cells

The aim of curing tumor is to eliminate tumors and preserve the organism as well as regain health. However, currently the chemotherapeutic cytotoxic kills both cancer cells and the normal with internecine result of damaging host cells, which is the heavily unreasonable contradiction between cytotoxic and suffers (or host cells). What should be done is to try to eliminate or resist the effect of killing normal cells and to research positively on intelligent anti-carcinomatous drugs with selectivity.

2. The contradiction between succession and discontinuity

It means the contradiction between the continuous divisions of cancer cells and the discontinuous chemotherapeutic period of treatment. The division and proliferation of cancer cells are continuous according to cell cycle, but chemotherapeutic drugs can be used with intervals for they inhibit the hematopoiesis of marrow and the blood corpuscle in the peripheral, which results in the severe contradiction between continuous divisions and proliferation of cancer cells and the discontinuous chemotherapies. Cancer cells divide successively, whereas chemotherapies are of interval, so cancer cells continue to divide during the intervals. Even a large dosage of chemotherapeutic drugs can only kill limited number of cancer cells, but can not destroy the whole. Even the majority of the cancer cells can be killed during the 3 to 5 days with chemotherapeutic drugs, the residual tumorous stem cells will continue to divide, to proliferate, to clone, and then metastasize and relapse when the effects of medicine fade away after several days. Therefore, killing cancer cells simply does not accord with the biological traits and behavior of cancer cells.

3. The contradiction between increase and decrease in immunity

That chemotherapeutic drugs usually can reduce the immunity contradicts the fact that the treatment on cancer should improve the immunity. As chemotherapeutic drugs can weaken the immunity, the longer the period of treatment, the more decrease in immunity, which promotes the decline in immunity, and even leads to lose monitor and the further development of tumors. This unreasonable contradiction between chemotherapy and immunity can weaken the curative effects heavily and even lead to diffuse. Therefore, treatment on tumors must aim at improving immunity and restoring immune monitor so as to stabilize the cancer, to make it and regain health.

4. **The contradiction between periods of treatment and curative effects**

That chemotherapy can inhibit marrow forces the peripheral leucocytes and blood platelets decline, so it is necessary to design the time of administering with intervals, which means the next time of chemotherapy should be taken on after restoration. Currently the intervals are just for waiting, instead of taking any measure to control cell division. On one hand cancer cells proliferate successively, on the other hand the chemotherapy stops. Due to this contradiction, it is difficult to gain the curative effects though chemotherapy. The more times of chemotherapy, the more serious immune inhibition will be, the more actively cancer cells proliferate during intervals, which results in evolution and metastasis during the process of chemotherapy.

5. **The contradiction between the period when drugs act and the cell cycle during the period of administer through intravenous drip**

It is only effective when the time of administer meets the sensitive cycle of cancer cells. If not, it is of no effect. Chemotherapeutic administer aims at cell cycles. During the period of administer, the cell cycles of most cancer cells in the crowds are not simultaneous but much different from each other, for instance, administer via intravenous drip from 8 am to 10 am when some of the cancer cells are in S stage, others are in G_1 or M stage. Thus, if the drug aims at S stage, it is effective to the cancer cells in S stage, but the drug given at this period (8 am to 10 am) is of no effect to the cancer cells in other stages, that is to say the sensitivity of chemotherapeutic drugs to cancer cells in different stages are differential. So during the period of administer through intravenous drip, it is effective to some sensitive cancer cells but not to those in insensitive periods.

6. **The contradiction between inhibition and protection of marrow**

Chemotherapy is cytotoxic and can inhibit the hematopiesis of marrow where hematopoietic stem cells are stored. Inhibition of marrow is a common clinical toxic reaction, which is the kinetic effect of chemotherapeutic drugs on specific stem cells. Chemotherapeutic cytotoxic drugs can damage the specific crowd of stem cells in marrow and will definitely reduce the number of mature and functional blood corpuscles in the peripheral blood. The degree of reduction relates to the lifetime of the cell components in the peripheral blood, for instance, the lifetime of hematid is longer, so the degree of reduction in the amount of blood corpuscles in the peripheral blood and the number of blood corpuscles in the peripheral blood during the treatment do not change obviously. However, the lifetimes of blood platelet and granular leucocytes are shorter with 3 days and 67 hours respectively, so the numbers of peripheral blood platelet and granular leucocytes reduce rapidly if the groups of megakaryocytic stem cells and granular cell groups are destroyed. If the amount of leucocytes and blood platelets decline to a very low level, it is extremely easy to cause subsequent serious infection or haemorrhage. In some cases, using large amount of broadspectrum antibiotic to resist the serious infection may lead to double infection or mycotic ingection, even endangers the life.

Authors: Xu Ze (China) ; Xu Jie(China) ; Bin Wu(America)

To sum up, in order to solve the contradictions in the current chemotherapy, to ameliorate its disadvantages and make it better, the author thinks that it is necessary to update thoughts and to research on new drugs and new principles to resist cancer and metastasis as well as relapse, except improving chemotherapy further in traditional thoughts, only the changes in the opinions on curing cancer and the creativities and reforms of technologies can bring further development into the treatment of cancer.

4

The initiative to change the solid body tumor intravenous chemotherapy into the target organ intravascular chemotherapy

- *Advocacy for traditional cancer therapies*
- *Assessment of problems and disadvantages of solid body tumor intravenous chemotherapy*
- *To change and perform the Intravascular chemotherapy into the target organ intravenous chemotherapy for solid tumors*
- *The initiative of specific methods and approaches of target organ intravascular chemotherapy of abdominal solid tumor*

The author reformed the systemic intravenous chemotherapy of solid tumor (especially the tumor of liver, gallbladder, pancreas, spleen, kidney, lung, uterus, ovary, abdominal cavity and pelvic cavity) to intravascular chemotherapy in target organ. This is the reformation after we have deeply taken cognizance of its disadvantages. Over the past half a century, millions of cancer patients have had chemotherapy and undertaken the side reaction of chemotherapy once and again after receiving the chemotherapy.

I. **Evaluation of Problems and Disadvantages of Systemic Intravenous Chemotherapy for Solid Tumor**

(I) **Evaluation of the route of administration of systemic intravenous chemotherapy for solid tumor**

The route of administration, not the specific targeting administration, distributes the cytotoxic drug in the whole body through the general blood circulation. In this way, it does not have a definite object for administration, but administers drugs in the whole body, resulting in:

1. The diseased cancer lesion area is very small (accounting for very small ratio of the body surface area of the whole body) only can obtain very little cytotoxic drug, resulting in very little action and curative effect.

2. However, the disease-free normal tissue in the whole body is damaged by the reaction of 99.6% of the cytotoxic drug. The normal tissue in the whole body does not need the cytotoxic drug, but it obtains a large number of cytotoxic drugs. However, the cytotoxic anti-cancer drug has relatively toxicity to the tissue with relatively rapid proliferation, such as the toxicity of alimentary canel, hemopoietic system, heart, liver, spleen, lung, kidney, nervous system and endocrine system, in this way, so many patients cannot receive the treatment or have to interrupt the treatment. Killing the tissue with relatively rapid proliferation in the whole body leads to harm to the patients instead of benefits to the patients.

3. The medication of this route of administration, does not have a definite object for administration, but the blind administration, which is non-targeting administration. Without the definite object, it only distributes and administers the drug in the whole body, as a result, the cancer lesion obtains a minute of cytotoxic drug while the area of the tissue in the whole body damaged by the cytotoxic drug is very large, resulting in bad curative effects, large side reaction and many and heavy complication, so the medication is unreasonable and unscientific.

4. With the above-mentioned medication, the cytotoxic drug administered in chemotherapy does not greatly attack the cancer cells, but only attach the cancer cells slightly (0.4%) while the normal tissue is greatly attacked in an all-round way by the cytotoxic drug (99.6%), at the same time, the cancer patient has low immunologic function by nature, now the cytotoxic drug in chemotherapy kills the hematopoietic cells, immunological cells, T lymphocyte, blood cells and blood platelet of the bone marrow again, resulting in further drop of immunologic function, the cytotoxic drug in chemotherapy attacks and kills the hematopoietic cells and immunological cells of the bone marrow once and again, resulting in the future drop of the immunologic function, in this way, one disaster comes after another, some cytotoxic drugs even urge the breakdown of the immunologic function.

(II) Elevation of calculation of dose for systemic intravenous chemotherapy for solid tumor

1. Since the systemic intravenous chemotherapy for solid tumor is not the specific targeting administration, but blindly distributed in the whole body, it necessarily needs much dose of cytotoxic drug; furthermore, it needs the combination of multiple drugs, in this way, it is possible to make the cancer lesion with very small area obtain the dose for remitting and shrinking the cancer lesion. The reason for large dose is that the 99.6% of the dose is absorbed by the whole body while only 0.4% is absorbed by the local cancer lesion. As a result, the relatively larger the dose, the larger and the more obvious the side reaction, resulting in remarkable drop of white blood cells and blood platelets, sometimes it also needs drug for increasing white cells, so it is unreasonable to calculate the dose.

2. At present, the systemic intravenous chemotherapy for solid tumor is the experience and the method obtained from the treatment of leukemia, however, as to the treatment

extended to the solid tumor, its guiding ideology is to administer the drug as per the calculation of the body surface area of the whole body, which is unadvisable. Why? Because the leukemic cells are distributed in the general blood circulation system, in the organs and tissues in the whole body, the target to be treated exists in the general blood circulation system, therefore, it is reasonable and advisable to adopt the systemic intravenous chemotherapy and conforms to the targeting treatment. Because the target cells of the leukaemia are distributed in the general blood circulation system, so it is reasonable and advisable. However, since the solid tumor is limited to a certain organ, its target to be treated is mainly a certain organ suffering from cancer, so it shall adopt the route of intravascular administration in the target organ and specific targeting administration, in this way, it can greatly reduce the dose of cytotoxic drug, as well as greatly reduce and eliminate the side reaction of the cytotoxic drug.

3. The calculation of the dose of systemic intravenous chemotherapy for solid tumor as per the body surface area is not based on therapeutical does by which how many cancer cells can be killed but on the tolerance dose of the organism to the cytotoxic drug. It is unknown whether one chemotherapy and two chemotherapies kill the cancer cells and how many cancer cells are killed by the chemotherapy. It is unknown. Whether there are cancer cells in the body of the patient? And where? It is unknown. Only one chemotherapy is carried out and only one task is accomplished.

(III) Evaluation of curative effect evaluation criterion of systemic intravenous chemotherapy for solid tumor

1. In a word, the curative effect evaluation criterion of systemic intravenous chemotherapy for solid is mainly embodied in three points: size of tumor, remission and remission time. As to the size of tumor, it is mainly based on CT, MRI or type-B ultrasonic, however, all of the images only reflect the size of occupation. As to the size of occupation, in our opinion, "the big" does not mean "the bad" and "the small" does not mean "the good". In addition, most of the occupations are short-term, the reason has been mentioned above.

2. Remission and remission time. Why the remission is regarded as the curative effect evaluation criterion and why the remission has a certain period? Apparently, the remission is not the objective of treatment or the treatment requirement of the patient or the objective of determination of treatment of the doctor just because the patient pays a certain price after several chemotherapies and only obtains a short-term remission. However, at present, the tumor medicine cannot heal all cancers (namely non-recurrence and non-metastasis) for a long time. Then, to say the latest, remission is better than the failure to remission. It is practical and realistic. Why it only can remit the cancer? Because the cytotoxic drug only harms the cancer cells and destroys their DNA rather than killing all cancer cells, which is only the first order kinetics. In addition, the reaction duration of cytotoxic drug only lasts 24h–48h even 72h after drug injection, after several days, the cancer cells will also be divided, proliferated and cloned in geometric progression, one

into two, two into four and four into eight. Since the cytotoxic drug cannot kill the stem cells of the tumor, after administration for chemotherapy, the stem cells of tumor are still divided, proliferated and cloned. So in out opinion, killing the cancer cells does not conform to biological characteristics and behaviors or multi-link and multi-step of the metastasis of cancer cells, it only can regulate and control the cancer cells and prevents their division, proliferation and clone rather than the simple killing.

(IV) **Evaluation of side reaction of systemic intravenous chemotherapy for solid tumor**

Why the side reaction is so large? Just because this kind of route of administration needs so much dose or has to adopt combined administration. In order to remit and shrink the cancer, it has to determine the tolerance dose of the patient as the dose, in this way, the reaction is necessarily large and the damage is large, the distribution mode of this kind of route of administration leads to large dose or combined administration, otherwise, it is difficult to realize the curative effect criterion of shrinkage, in fact, it is avoidable to administer 99.6% of the cytotoxic drug to the normal tissues, in other words, it is avoidable to reform this route of administration to the specific targeting administration. If it is reformed to intravascular administration in the specific target organ, naturally, the side reaction will become little or be eliminated.

II. We Propose to Reform Systemic Intravenous Chemotherapy for Solid Tumor to Intravascular Chemotherapy in Target Organ

Since the above-mentioned problems are in existence, they shall be further studied. We should continue to improve the traditional curative therapeutic method as per the traditional idea, in the meanwhile, we should update the idea and the understanding, make progress in reforming and have the courage to innovate. Innovation, must challenge the traditional idea instead of replacement, it shall overcome the disadvantages, correct the defects so as to make it more perfect. Innovation, shall open a new path to overcome the cancer. Therefore, we specially propose the new idea, new concept and new principles of anti-cancer as well as new treatment mode and adopt organic integral new treatment mode to reform and innovate the traditional problems based on the biological characteristics and behaviors of cancer as well as the immunologic conditions of the host and the multi-link and multi-step of metastasis.

(I) **Necessity, reasonableness and scientificalness of reform the systemic intravenous chemotherapy for solid tumor to intravascular chemotherapy in target organ**

1. As above-mentioned, the route of administration of systemic intravenous chemotherapy is not the specific targeting administration but the blind general distribution, which is unreasonable and scientific distribution, so it must be reformed. The cancer lesion is limited to the local of the viscera, so it is necessary to adopt the specific targeting

administration with clear target, which is reasonable and scientific. As to the systemic intravenous chemotherapy, since most of the cytotoxic drugs are administered to the general normal tissues, if the drugs are administered to the target organ, it can save the dose administered to the whole body, in this way, the dose can be greatly reduced, thus the side reaction is greatly reduced even eliminated, so the chemotherapy even may have no toxicity.

2. Analyze the source and formation of the side reaction of chemotherapy and probe into the method to eliminate the side reaction. Through review, reflection and analysis, we deeply realize that the source, the blind distribution of the cytotoxic drug in the whole body by the systemic intravenous chemotherapy for solid tumor, is unreasonable. In order to shrink the tumor, it necessarily increases the dose, resulting in unavoidable side reaction.

The increased dose of cytotoxic drug does not entirely react on the cancer lesion, but mainly on the whole body to damage the normal histiocytes while these general normal tissues do not need the cytotoxic drug, however, they get most of the cytotoxic drugs in fact, which is unreasonable. It is necessary to study and reform it.

In view that its source and formation is based on the blindness of the route of administration of systemic intravenous chemotherapy, resulting in increased dose and combined administration and leading to unavoidable side reaction, so the solution is to reform the route of administration.

How to reform the route of administration?

Professor Xu Ze proposes to reform the systemic intravenous chemotherapy for solid tumor (especially the tumor of liver, gallbladder, spleen, pancreas, stomach, intestine, uterus, ovary, pelvic cavity and abdominal cavity) to intravascular chemotherapy in target organ, in this way, the drug is administered to the specific target and then to the cancer lesion of the target organ, necessarily leading in the greatly decreased dose; the reduction of dose of cytotoxic drug necessarily leads to the reduction and elimination of side reaction. The elimination of side reaction of the traditional chemotherapy, makes millions of cancer patients free from the pains and risks of side reaction of chemotherapy and benefits the patients.

Professor Xu Ze holds: the intravascular administration in the specific target organ, reduces the dose, improves the curative effects, eliminates the side reaction, necessarily leading to great reduction of medical charge, saving billions of medical charges and expenditures (in RMB Yuan) for the state and the patients and being advantageous for settling the problems of being difficult and expensive in taking medical treatment.

Over half a century, millions of cancer patients have been deeply damaged by the side reaction of the chemotherapy, therefore, this reform will benefit millions of cancer cells, which is a great pioneering undertaking and an original innovation and promotes the further development of the oncology in the 21st century.

(II)   **It is necessary to firstly study and make clear where the target is so as to carry out the intravascular chemotherapy in target organ; it is necessary to study and make clear where the cancer cells are so as to kill the cancer cells with cytotoxic drug in chemotherapy? In this way, it can have a definite object.**

1.   The primary lesion of the solid tumor is in the organ, for example, the stomach cancer lies in the stomach, the liver cancer lies in the liver, the lung cancer lies in the lung, the intestinal cancer lies in intestine, that is to say, the primary cancer lesion lies in the organ, even if it meets with metastasis in the advanced stage, its primary cancer lesion is still in the organ.

2.   Where are the cancer cells? The cancer cells of stomach cancer, intestinal cancer, liver cancer, lung cancer and so on are mainly in the portal system and meet with metastasis via the portal system. An example of liver cancer: the main blood supply of liver cancer is from the hepatic artery, the most primary route of the metastasis of liver cancer is the venous system in the liver. The metastasis of liver cancer in liver is the most common metastasis mode, the cancer cells invade the branch of the portal vein, form the cancer embolus in the portal vein, continually extend to the hepatic portal until the left and right branch of the portal vein and its beam are blocked by the cancer embolus, the deciduous cancer cell balls are floating in the portal vein and are spread to the liver through blood.

The hepatic vein wall is thin and receives the blood flowing back from the cancer lesion, so it is easy to be encroached and the cancer embolus is formed in the hepatic vein, sometimes, the embolus can reach to inferior vena cava and to right atrium and then meet with metastasis via the lung.

The liver is one of the organs meeting with metastatic carcinoma most commonly. According to information of pathologic anatomy, among the cases of the patients who die of the malignant tumor, about 40% meet with the liver metastasis and its incidence rate is next only to lymphatic system. The liver metastasis of malignant tumor of gstrointestinal tract is the most common.

The liver receives the dual blood supply from portal vein and hepatic artery, the liver metastasis can come from the portal vein circulation and systemic circulation, that is to say, the cancer cells enters the systemic circulation via pulmonary capilliary station. The blood supply is complicated, about 90%of the blood supply is from the hepatic artery.

3.   The administration along the route of hematogenous metastasis of cancer cells for tracking and killing shall follow the flow direction of the tumor vein, the chemotherapy drug follows the flow direction, killing the cancer cells in metastasis with small dose. As to the cancer cells, the cancer cell groups and micro-metastasis cancer embolus in metastasis, it is only necessary to kill $10^{4.5}$ cancer cells with eth cytotoxic drugs for

chemotherapy, the rest $10^{4.5}$ cancer cells can be eliminated by the immunological cells and immunological surveillance in the blood circulation of the organism. According to the plan, it is satisfactory for the dose to kill $10^{4.5}$ cancer cells, the dose cannot go so far to kill too many immunological cells. To kill some cancer cells and to protect the immunological cells from being damaged excessively as well, shall be judged with the sign of not affecting the drop of white blood cells and blood platelets. The viscera and organs in the abdomen, such as stomach, rectum, colon, liver, gallbladder, pancreas, uterus and ovary and other tumor-producing vein gather at the portal vein system, therefore, the target organs of tumor at the abdomen shall focus on the portal vein system and hepatic artery.

III. **Xu Ze Proposes to Reform the Systemic Intravenous Chemotherapy for Solid Tumor at the Abdomen to the Specific Method and Approach of Intravascular Chemotherapy in Target Organ**

(I) **Intravascular administration for chemotherapy in target organ**

1. Administration via arterial route

    (1) The chemotherapy pump shall be arranged in the hepatic artery;
    (2) Hepatic artery interventional therapy, embolism + chemotherapy;
    (3) Interventional chemotherapy perfusion of bronchial artery;
    (4) Interventional chemotherapy perfusion of internal iliac artery;
    (5) Interventional chemotherapy of arteria pancreatica;
    (6) Interventional chemotherapy perfusion of gastric artery;
    (7) Hepatic artery chemotherapy pump through laparotomy.

2. Administration via portal vein route

    (1) Portal vein chemotherapy pump through laparotomy;
    (2) Omentum venous pump through laparotomy;
    (3) Subcutaneous chemotherapy pump through laparotomy via mesentery vein;
    (4) Subcutaneous deep vein conduit chemotherapy pump: can be used in the treatment of malignant tumor of the intestines and stomach tract.

    Surgical interventional chemotherapy for tumor patient has been widely applied, now the subcutaneous chemotherapy pump for drug delivery system is mostly adopted at present and it is a good route of administration for tumor chemotherapy, which can be divided into three classes: venous duct chemotherapy pump; ductus arteriosus chemotherapy pump and celiac duct chemotherapy pump, compared with the peripheral vein chemotherapy and artery interventional chemotherapy, it has a lot of advantages.

3.   Administration via target organ at the abdomen

Oral administration: oral administration→ stomach→ vena coronaria of stomach (left vein and right vein of stomach)→ splenic vein→ portal vein, for example, oral administration of Xeloda.

Oral administration: oral administration→ stomach→ lymphatic vessel under gastric mucosa →lymph node around the stomach→ lymph node behind peritoneum→ cisterna chyli→ thoracic duct, for example, oral administration of Brucea emulsion.

Rectal suppository: rectal suppository (a few of chemotherapy drug) → venae intestinales → vein under mesentery → portal vein.

Route of administration for the target organ of lung cancer:

A.   vein of antibrachium → superior vena cava → double lungs
B.   Portal vein conduit or pump → liver → hepatic vein →lower caval vein → right ventricle → double lungs
C.   Oral administration: oral administration → portal vein →liver →lower caval vein → right ventricle → double lungs

(II)   Paying attention to arterial interventional administration

An example of liver cancer: since the onset of liver cancer is insidious, when the patient see a doctor, it is mostly in intermediate and advanced stage, followed by other factors such as high combined hepatocirrhosis rate, relatively low surgical removal rate and high recurrence rate after operation, most of the patients need non-operation therapy. At present, among the non-operation therapies with positively curative effects, interventional therapy is most widely used.

Its indication can be used to the liver cancer in different stages and it is better for the liver cancer in early and intermediate stage. These suffering from serious icterrus, voluminous ascites, serious damage to liver function and widespread metastasia shall be abstained from contraindication.

Generally, the first period of treatment of interventional therapy of liver cancer needs 3-4 times, with the interval of 2-3 months. In principle, the next interventional therapy shall be carried out only after the general condition and liver function of the patient are basically recovered over 3 weeks.

Interventional therapy

Since the interventional therapy will damage the normal tissue especially the liver and the immune system of the organism synchronously, the organism needs a certain time for recovery to understand the second interventional therapy, in the interval of interventional therapy, it shall nourish the liver, improve the immunity and adopt the complex treatment. In Shuguang Tumor Clinic of Shugang Tumor Research Institute, in the past 16 years, all the patients of liver cancer receiving the interventional therapy administer XZ-C medicine after operation and they take oral administration of XZ-C$_{1+4+5}$ for protecting the chest, improving the immunity, protecting the bone marrow, enhancing hematopiesis, protecting liver and great curative effects have been made. Most of the patients have been in good condition and have had good appetite, their symptoms have been improved, their survival quality has been improved, and most of them have had an obviously prolonged survival period.

(III) Paying attention to the route of administration of chemotherapy pump in portal vein

It is necessary for the specific targeting administration for target organ to understand where the target organ of the cancer cells is. The tumor-bearing vein of stomach cancer, colon and rectal cancer, gallbladder cancer, pancreas cancer, cancer of pelvic cavity and oophoroma flows into the portal vein system, therefore, the cancer cells, and the ones in metastasis are flowing into the portal vein system, therefore, attention shall be paid to the chemotherapy pump in portal vein for targeting tracking and killing the cancer cells.

Chemotherapy pump in portal vein is remained in the portal vein after exploration of laparotomy or remained in the lower omentum vein after laparotomy; or remained in the drug delivery system in the mesentery under the direct vision of the laparotomy.

Chemotherapy pump embedded in portal vein body, also called implanted drug delivery system or subcutaneous embedded drug delivery system, is a kind of drug subcutaneously embedded for local perfusion, which is used for the guiding chemotherapy of cancer and oriented local perfusion chemotherapy for preventing the recurrence after removal of tumor. The drug can directly enter the target organ through drug pump and conduit, improving the lethality and the curative effects to cancer cells and reducing the side reaction of chemotherapy. It is reported by the literature that when the density of the local chemotherapy drug is increased one time, the lethality to the tumor can be increased 6-12 times. This system can increase several times of the density of the local drug. At present, this system is widely used for the clinic at home and abroad and great curative effects have been made.

In a word, as above mentioned, the systemic intravenous chemotherapy for solid tumor, only has a few of drug reaching to the cancer lesion while most of the cytotoxic drugs react on the normal histiocyte in the whole body, especially, they are relatively toxic to the tissue with rapid proliferation such as hemopoietic system of bone marrow, immune system and alimentary system and have the side reaction, however, these normal tissue, not needing the cytotoxic drugs, obtains a large number of cytotoxic drugs, which is unreasonable.

As to the chemotherapy through intravascular administration in the target organ, the drug is directly sent to the target organ via the conduit, the cytotoxic drugs obtained by the cancer lesion are all drugs administered, which is reasonable and scientific, greatly reducing the dose for chemotherapy. The specific targeting administration, reduces the does, improves the curative effects, reduces or eliminates the side reaction. In this way, it improves the curative effects, eliminates the reaction, resulting in the reduction of expenses. It is advantages for settling the problems of being difficult and expensive in taking medical treatment. Since it reduces or eliminates the side reaction, necessarily reducing the medical charge and saving billions of medical expenses and expenditures (in RMB Yuan) for the state.

This topic is my third book "new concept of cancer treatment and a new method," the core of the twelfth chapter, this article advocates "on the solid tumor systemic intravenous chemotherapy should be the target organ for intravascular chemotherapy"

Why is this initiative?

Because half a century, the size of the world's hospitals in all countries to buy body tumors are using systemic intravenous chemotherapy, the hospital tumor chemotherapy are busy patients with systemic intravenous chemotherapy, cancer patients are also hospitalized for intravenous chemotherapy, the above Through our in-depth measurement found and commented on the existence of systemic intravenous chemotherapy problems and disadvantages,

In this paper, we put forward this: a review of solid body intravenous chemotherapy route of the drawbacks of the second assessment of solid body tumor intravenous chemotherapy dose calculation; three evaluation of solid tumor systemic intravenous chemotherapy efficacy evaluation criteria ; Four assessment of solid body tumor intravenous chemotherapy side effects. Since the discovery of the existence of the problem, it should try to improve, how to improve, how to reform?

First of all to study the patient's cancer cells where? Through our laboratory for many years of animal experimental research and clinical research found that abdominal surgery, gastrointestinal cancer patients with cancer cells are homogeneous in the portal vein system, the abdomen of various metastases to the liver metastases of cancer cells are also cancer Into the hepatic portal vein or hepatic vein, we found in surgery is also true.

Therefore, we advocate should be reformed for the portal vein system drug pump, change the body of the drug distribution for the target organ administration, the target clear, directly to the chemical drug by the drug pump directly to the portal vein system, direct contact with the presence of portal vein cancer cells The In my nearly 10 years follow-up cases, the portal vein system to set the pump long-term effect is better, in this paper, I put forward specific programs and methods.

The reform of the hospital on the National Academy of Oncology will cause a huge shock and change the current national hospitals of the Department of Chemists doctors, on the daily work is to make the whole body intravenous chemotherapy venous puncture, observation care, if the reform For the portal vein to set the pulp, the soil to be carried out by the surgeon, rather than chemotherapy doctors and nurses involved, involving a series of reforms, changes. For half a century, tens of thousands of solid tumor cancer patients around the world have undergone systemic intravenous chemotherapy, drug body distribution, but so far cancer is still the first death, and can not prevent recurrence and metastasis.

In this paper, this solid tumor intravenous chemotherapy route of the proposed challenge, challenge, criticism and reform, will be possible to correct the change over half a century to the whole body of intravenous chemotherapy to the irrational status quo. (The above are our first in the international, independent innovation, the international leader.)

In the last two centuries, the treatment of malignant tumors has occurred twice leap:

The first time was 1890 Naistad proposed the concept of radical surgery.

The first time in the 1970s, Fish integrated chemotherapy into radical surgery (adjuvant chemotherapy or neoadjuvant chemotherapy).

Since then, the treatment of malignant tumors wandering.

Fish is the route of systemic intravenous chemotherapy, after half a day, so far failed to reduce the mortality rate also failed to prevent the hair, transfer, mortality is still the first. Now we are on this traditional doctrine, the traditional method of questioning and reforming the idea of innovation, instead of target organ administration, combined with the establishment of xz-c comprehensive treatment concept and xz-c immunomodulation therapy (ie immunotherapy) will be helpful To promote the current situation of the current hovering.

5

Initiatives to strategies of improving cancer postoperative adjuvant chemotherapy

- *Why should cancer postoperative adjuvant chemotherapy be performed ?*
- *The analysis of reasons why Postoperative chemotherapy did not meet the desired*
- *how to do cancer postoperative adjuvant chemotherapy well*

Since 1990s, in view that the reoccurrence and metastasis rate of cancer after operation was very high, in order to prevent the reoccurrence and metastasis after operation, a series of assistance chemotherapy after operation has been adopted, what's more, the chemotherapy was made before operation (for example, the breast cancer), however, the results had been not so satisfactory. Reoccurrence and metastasis take place in assistant chemotherapy after operation or in the period of treatment or the metastasis takes place synchronously in chemotherapy. It can be seen from so many patients in Wuhan Shuguang Tumor Special Clinic that neither reoccurrence nor metastasis cannot be prevented by the assistant chemotherapy after operation, even in some cases, the intensified chemotherapy promotes the adynamia of immunologic function. All these things should be seriously, calmly, practically and realistically thought and reflected by the clinicians: why the assistant chemotherapy after operation cannot prevent the reoccurrence? Why the assistant chemotherapy after operation cannot prevent the metastasis? Why the assistant chemotherapy after operation on some patients promotes the adynamia of immunologic function? What's the problem and disadvantage of the assistant chemotherapy after operation? What measures should be taken? How to further study and perfect it? How to reform and innovate in the assistant chemotherapy to improve the curative effects?

I. **Why to make the assistant chemotherapy after operation on cancer or assistant chemotherapy in peri-operation period?**

Currently, the treatment of cancer mainly depends on the operation, however, the reoccurrence and metastasis rate is still relatively high after operation.

1. **The potential reason why the local reoccurrence and metastasis after radical operation on cancer takes place may be the following factors viewed from clinic:**

(1)   Insufficient attention has not been paid to the free-tumor technique, as a result, the operation such as exploration and touch causes the cancer cells on the serosa surface to fall into the intra-abdominal implantation.

(2)   The tumor tissue is not thoroughly removed by the operation, as a result, the remained cancer cells are continually proliferating.

(3)   The existing metastasis lesion is not found in operation and is not removed, for example, the lymph node in metastasis is not found or is removed incompletely.

(4)   As to the clearing of lymph node in operation, traditionally, it adopts the passive separation, in this way, the apocoptic micro-lymphatic vessel may lead to the fluxion, dissemination, residual and transplantation of the cancer cells.

(5)   The operation leads to the transplantation of the cancer cells, the cancer cells invading the esophagus, stomach serosa or colon, recta and serosa may easily fall into the abdominal cavity and form the transplantation lesion and the damaged peritoneum in the area of operation may easily meet with transplnation and reoccurrence. The reoccurrence of anastomotic stoma of the colon may be the intracavity exfoliation and transplantation of the enteral cancer cells in the operation.

(6)   The metastasis of the lymph node in the patients in the late stage is relatively wide and syzygial, in this way, it is difficult to remove it with operation.

(7)   In the operation on gastrointestinal tract cancer, the metastasis of cancer cells in the portal vein takes place, resulting in the metastasis of liver cancer cells after operation. However, it is unseenable in the operation by the naked eyes. For example, when the "radical operation on gastric carcinoma" is made, the cancerous protuberance and the tumid lymph nodes of gastric carcinoma can be seen by us, however, whether the cancer cells exist in the vein and the blood of the portal vein is unknown? How many cancer cells exist? Where do these cancer cells in the vein go? Whether these cancer cells in cluster that can be touched and extruded into the venous blood in operation arrive at the portal vein? Or arrive at the branch of the portal vein in the liver? It is not impossible to touch the cancerous protuberance in exploration and excision of gastric cancerous protuberance and cleaning of lymph node, the operation necessarily makes a large number of cancer cells be extruded and fall down, then they flow into the portal venous blood, resulting in metastasis in liver after operation.

(8)   The operation brings about the traumas to the organism, resulting in the inferior immunologic function, in this way, the organism losses the immunological surveillance or is weakened in immunological surveillance, leaving opportunity to the residual cancer cells or the cancer cells in dormancy for reoccurrence and metastasis.

(9)   As to the cancer in the progressive stage, the metastasis of cancer cells may take place before operation while these cancer cells in metastasis cannot be seen by the

physician in operation. However, it is reported in the pathological section report that the cancer embolus can be seen in the blood capillary and the lymphatic vessel.

Based on the above-mentioned, after the radical operation of the cancer, the residual cancer cells may still exist, resulting in reoccurrence and metastasis of the residual subclinical cancer lesion after operation.

Then, how to make up for the shortage of radical operation with residual cancer cells? Adopt the chemotherapy in peri-operation period to hunt the residual cancer cells in operation with the chemotherapy cytotoxic drug and remove the cancer cells falling off or remained or transplanted in the operation.

However, could the traditional assistant chemotherapy after operation hunt the residual cancer cells in operation? Could it remove the cancer cells falling off, remained or transplanted in operation?

2. **Why the current assistant chemotherapy after operation cannot prevent the reoccurrence and metastasis? It shall be reviewed, analyzed and reflected:**

(1) The route of administration of assistant chemotherapy after operation shall be further studied and reformed. At present, it mainly adopts the general intravenous chemotherapy after operation, the cytotoxic drug injected is generally distributed, acting on the histiocytes of the viscera in the whole body, in this way, the ones killed are mainly the proliferative cells, immunological cells and bone marrow cells of the normal tissue organs in the whole body. However, the field of operation accounts for a little ratio in the whole body, in this way, the dose obtained is very small, it is difficult to kill the local residual cancer cells or the cancer lesion in the field of operation or the residual cancer lesion of the cancer cells falling off in the operation, therefore, the route of administration shall be reformed.

(2) The assistant chemotherapy after operation is blinded and the drug administered is not subject to the drugsensitive test. Since the drugsensitive test on the cancer histiocytes of patient is not carried out, the drug is administered by experience, so it is unknown whether the drug is sensitive. If the drug administered is insensitive or drug resistant, it is not only fruitless, without any action on the residual cancer cells, but also kills the proliferative cells, the immunological cells and the bone marrow cells of the normal tissues in the whole body, while these normal tissues in the whole body do not need the cytotoxic drug, resulting in the remarkable side effect, damaging the patient and making the patient suffer from the pain of the side effect. Thus, although the chemotherapy has been made for several times, the expected curative effects cannot be realized, in addition, the cytotoxic drug injected intravenously in the wholly body covers the whole body, kills the general immunological cells and the hematopoietic cells of the bone marrow and makes the immunologic functions of the patient further descend. Actually, the cancer patient is inferior in immunologic function, while the radical operation further brings

down the immunologic function, plus the assistant chemotherapy of the cytotoxic drug after operation, the immunological function of the patient is further reduced, like one disaster after another, resulting in metastasis while in chemotherapy. Therefore, as for the assistant chemotherapy after operation, if the drugsensitive test is not made and the drug is administered in form of individualization, the chemotherapy would benefit some patients while damage some patients.

(3) Assistant chemotherapy after operation. **Since the tumor is removed and the lymph clearing is made, the drug administration plan and the dosage should differ from the ones for the patients without removal by operation,** the dosage in the assistant chemotherapy period after operation would differ from the one before operation, before removal of the tumor, the dosage is calculated as per the body surface area so as to realize the goal of remission and shrinkage, however, after the radical operation, the tumor is removed, so it shall target the potentially residual cancer cells or the micro-metastasis in operation instead of the remission and shrinkage, since both targets differs from each other, in order to remit and shrink the tumor of the patient without operation, the drug must have a certain lethality, as a result, the drug administration plans shall be combined and the dosage shall be up to the one the patient can bear, in this way, the curative effect of remission and shrinkage can be realized. Meanwhile, the assistant chemotherapy after operation, depends on radical operation primarily and the chemotherapy secondarily, only targeted for removal of the potentially residual cancer cells or the cancer cells falling off in the operation or the cancer cells in metastasis to make some subsidiary treatment to prevent the reoccurrence and metastasis. Therefore, its drug administration plan and dose shall differ from the former and the dosage of the cytotoxic drug shall be greatly reduced.

(4) What determines the indications and the contraindications of the assistant chemotherapy after operation? At present, the indications of assistant chemotherapy after operation are discordant, for example, do the residual cancer cells exist in the patient after this operation on earth? Where? How many? To what extent? All those things should be taken into account and estimated, however, most of the patients receive the "radical operation on cancer" in the general surgery or the specialized surgery, after operation, they come back to the local hospitals or the tumor clinic, the chemotherapy after operation is the general intravenous chemotherapy, the plans selected differ from each other in each place, each hospital by each physician, namely there is no uniform plan, these physicians or nurses responsible for general intravenous injection for the assistant chemotherapy after operation are not always aware of the patient's condition, pathological analysis, the range and the extent of cancer invasion seen in the operation as well as the estimation of the potential residual cancer lesion in operation, the extent of the radical operation and so on. They should know TNM stage and the immunity chemotherapy and estimate the potential residual cancer cells. Who knows it

clearly? Only the operation doctor because he can see the range and extent of the cancer invasion through exploration in operation. Therefore, what determines the selection of chemotherapy or radiotherapy after operation? The operation physician shall determine the indications and the contraindications of the assistant chemotherapy after operation as well as the chemotherapy plan, times, dosage and so on to satisfy the actual conditions of the patient.

(5) How to assess the curative effects of the assistant chemotherapy after operation? At present, there is no uniform understanding or standard. The objective curative effects of the chemotherapy on the solid tumor before removal of the tumor shall be assessed according to the area of tumor and the remission of the tumor recognized in the world. However, since the tumor is removed, it shall be assessed according to the improvement of the symptom and the condition instead of area of tumor. At present, what role does the assistant chemotherapy after operation play? Does it kill the cancer cells? How many? Do the residual cancer cells exist in the patient's body? What is the effect? All these things are kept unknown. However, it is well known that it kills the normal cells, the immunological cells and the hematopoietic cells of the bone marrow because the white blood cells fall down, the blood platelets fall down too, but it is the extent of the side effect rather than the effect. As to the tumor sign, it is difficult to determine the definite standard at present and it is necessary to make the fundamental study and clinical study.

II. the analysis of the reasons why postoperative chemotherapy did not meet expectations

After more than 10 years, postoperative adjuvant chemotherapy has been carried out in factories across the country.

However, most of the postoperative adjuvant chemotherapy is based on experience alone. The treatment regimes vary from place to place, and the chemotherapeutic drugs used are different. The same hospital has different departments and doctors because of different experiences.

The number of chemotherapy drugs and the number of days in the interval are slightly different in each hospital. There are 1 person per month, and there are 2 people every 2 months, once a week, 4 times in a row. For 6 consecutive times, there are 8 consecutive times or even 10 times. The treatment settings have greater blindness and are different; the choice of the program and the choice of drugs have a certain blindness, and they are also different, and there is no uniform or consistent standardization standard. Because most hospitals did not conduct drug susceptibility testing, they failed to achieve "individualized" chemotherapy.

The current postoperative adjuvant chemotherapy regimen is basically similar to the usual chemotherapy regimen, but the usual chemotherapy target or "target" of the tumor is for primary or metastatic cancer, and the therapeutic target is to make the primary cancer mass, Metastatic cancer masses or enlarged lymph nodes shrink, disappear, and alleviate. These solid tumors have a large volume. If you want to reduce them, you must use a large number of chemotherapy drugs, otherwise it is difficult to reach the mouth.

However, postoperative adjuvant chemotherapy is completely different from this because radical surgery removes the swollen lymph nodes from the primary tumor and surrounding areas without a solid tumor. Since the cancer block has been resected, the purpose of postoperative adjuvant chemotherapy is mainly for cancer cells, micrometastasis or cancer cells that may be metastasized after surgery, with the goal of targeting residual or potentially metastatic cancer cells instead of For tumor entities, the dose should be small and does not damage or minimally damage the host's immune cells.

Therefore, to evaluate the efficacy of postoperative adjuvant chemotherapy, it can not be measured by whether the tumor is reduced, but whether it improves immunity, improves the quality of life, improves symptoms, raises immune index, reduces tumor markers, and spirit. As with the appetite situation, etc. as the evaluation criteria.

III. how to do postoperative adjuvant chemotherapy for cancer

The author proposed the following improvements and development suggestions for postoperative adjuvant chemotherapy for abdominal cancer (malignant tumors such as liver, gallbladder, pancreas, stomach, intestine, and abdominal cavity).

1. Reform the route of administration and change the general intravenous chemotherapy into the chemotherapy through intravascular administration in target organ. All of the operations on cancer in abdomen, no matter the radical operation or palliative excision, or the operation only for exploration instead of removal, shall adopt the built-in pump in ductus venosus in stomach omentum, or built-in pump in portal vein, or arterial pump, or built-in pump in vein of mesentery as much as possible. Why is the chemotherapy pump built in portal system? Firstly, it is necessary to know where the cancer cells after operation on cancer exist. The administration must be targeted for the cancer cell group and the cancer cells of liver cancer, gallbladder cancer, pancreatic cancer, gastric cancer and intestinal cancer are in the tuberiferous veins, which flow towards the portal vein and gather at the portal vein, then flow towards hepatic vein via sinus hepaticus and into the lungs via the right atrium. Therefore, the portal system adopts the targeted intravascular administration targeted through the chemotherapy pump, so it is the direct target and it is reasonable and scientific. It can make the residual cancer cells prowling in the portal vein after operation directly contact the chemotherapy drug to produce the curative effect.

2. Reform the dosage of administration: since the built-pump in portal vein is directly targeted for the cancer cell group in the blood of the portal vein and the chemotherapy drug needed is greatly reduced by contrast with the dosage of general intravenous administration. Since the drug is administered through the target organ of the portal vein, the dosage can be greatly reduced. Because the radical operation on cancer has been made, the cancerous protuberance has been removed and the next thing to be done is to remove the potentially residual cancer cells, generally, the immunological cells in the human body can remove these cancer cells, however, since the immunologic function of the cancer patient comes down, the assistant chemotherapy after operation is used to assist in removal, so only a small quantity of dosage

is needed, it shall strive for killing 10^{5-6} cancer cells without damage to the normal cells as much as possible. The rest 10^{5-6} cancer cells will be removed by the immunological cells of the organism. However, as to the tracking and hunting of the potential cancer cells in metastasis in the portal system, although the targeted administration reduces the dosage greatly, the drug concentration in the portal vein will be greatly increased out of question, resulting in the improvement of the curative effect. **Since the dosage is greatly reduced, it will necessarily reduce even eliminate the side effect of the chemotherapy greatly. The elimination of the side effect of the chemotherapy, will benefit millions of cancer patients. Over the past half century, millions of cancer patients have deeply suffered from the pain of the side effect from the chemotherapy and the radiotherapy all over the world, what's more, the lives of some patients have been endangered. Since the side effect of chemotherapy is eliminated, so many cancer patients are secured. The cancer seriously endangers the health of the human beings and makes the medical expenses rapidly increase as well. The direct expenses for cancer treatment in China are approximately RMB one hundred billion Yuan, bringing a heavy economic burden to the patients even the whole society. Now Professor Xu Ze holds: the intravascular administration in the specific target organ, reduces the dose, improves the curative effects, eliminates the side reaction, necessarily leading to great reduction of medical charge, saving billions of medical charges and expenditures (in RMB Yuan) for the state and the patients and being advantageous for settling the problems of being difficult and expensive in taking medical treatment.**

3. Reform the blindness of the drug administered for assistant chemotherapy after operation. The drug for chemotherapy after operation shall be subject to the drugsensitive test together with the histiocytes of the cancer tissue of the patients for the individualized chemotherapy. All operations on cancer, no matter the radical operations or the palliative operations or the exploratory operations, shall try to obtain the specimen of the cancer tissue, the cancer tissue will be cut up into two halves in aseptic manipulation, one for cultivation of cancer tissue and drugsensitive test and another for pathological section and chemotherapy of immunity group for definite pathological diagnosis.

Why the specimen of cancer tissue is selected for cultivation of cancer cells and the drugsensitive test? Since the detection of sensitivity and drug resistance of tumor chemotherapy is the foundation of "individualized" chemotherapy. To this day, the tumor chemotherapy has stridden forward to the "individualized" chemotherapy. In the past days, the different tumor patients receive the same chemotherapy mode (plan), resulting in blindness inevitably. It is shown by the study that the same kind of tumor with the same tissue, even the same tumor in different stages has the incompletely consistent sensitivity to the chemotherapy drug. Therefore, it is necessary to make the drugsensitive test on the tumor patient to select the sensitive drug. Especially, with the increase of the anti-tumor drug at present, it is more urgent. It is proven by the clinical experience in tumor chemotherapy that the effective rate of drug administered by experience is very low (14%) while it will be increased to 28%-35% if the results measured with the existing drugsensitive test method is used to guide the selection of the drug, which is a great fruit.

The detection of the sensitivity and drug resistance of tumor chemotherapy offers an important basis to the foreseeable chemotherapy to reasonably use the anti-tumor drug to reduce the blindness and improve the pertinence, which would undoubtedly improve the level of tumor chemotherapy greatly.

4. The key is to manage and disposal the pump after operation: the drug pump for portal system is in-built in the operation. After operation, it is necessary to continually adopt the long-term light (trace) nontoxic chemotherapy drug and inject the heparin to prevent the embolism, prevent the cancer embolus and prevent the cancer cell group. Where are the cancer cells in the peri-operation period? The cancerous protuberance of liver, gallbladder, pancreas, spleen, stomach and intestine will be carried off by the blood separately after flowing into the blood of the portal vein or many cancer cells meet with homoplasmic adhesion or heterogenetic adhesion with other cells to form the cancer cell group, which floats with the blood and forms the cancer embolus in the blood vessel, then the deciduous cancer cell embolus moves along the direction of the blood of the venous system. The cancer cells continually enter the blood circulation and transfer along the normal direction of the blood. Most of the cancer cells entering the blood circulation will be eliminated by the host and only a few of the cancer cells survive. Within several days after operation, a large number of cancer cells flow over into the portal system via tumorigenic vein in virtue of operation technique and exploratory extrusion. The surviving cancer cells are adhered to the endothelial cells of the wall of the target organ and then enter the target organ after passing through the wall and form the minute metastasis lesion. The cancer cells from gstrointestinal tract can flow into the liver along the portal vein and the liver is the end point of the blood of the portal vein, therefore, the cancer of gastrointestinal tract often transfers to the liver, forms the cancer cells of the metastasis lesion of the metastasis liver cancer and invades the central vein via the minute branch of the portal vein. The cancer cells can enter the hepatic vein and then flow back to the right atrium via the lower caval vein, then to the lung via the pulmonary artery and form the metastasis lesion of lung.

It can be often seen that the cancer embolus exists in the portal vein branch in the pathological report or the cancer embolus forms in the portal vein branch in CT or MRI report. The cancer embolus is the main factor in the formation of the metastasis lesion. The cancer cells, the fibrin and the blood platelet constitute the embolus and then it is carried to other parts, passes through the wall and forms the secondary tumor around the blood vessel. The formation of cancer embolus is related to the following factors: ① the inherent adhesion and aggregation of the cancer cells; ② the action of Thrombo-Pletinlike substances; ③ action of blood platelet; ④combined action of fibrin.

It is important to do well in management and application of pump after operation. Someone is inbuilt with chemotherapy pump and does not pay a return visit or use the pump after leaving hospital. After operation, the regular return visit shall be paid and the heparin shall be injected via the pump to prevent the blockade and the cancer embolus. A few of chemotherapy drugs shall be injected to hunt the floating cancer cells remaining in the the blood circulation of portal vein.

The surgeons and the nurses shall be responsible for the arrangement, follow-up survey, registration, filling, consultation answer, statistics and summary of the assistant chemotherapy after operation.

3. **Reform the single goal of killing cancer cells into the immunological mediation and control therapy in an all-round way.**

Abandon the goal of only killing the cancer cells, **attach importance to the resistance of the organism**, reform it into the immunological mediation and control therapy in an all-round way and give attention to both of them, thus, the curative effect will be improved. XZ-C medicine shall be orally taken in the period of assistant chemotherapy after operation and after the treatment course of the assistant chemotherapy to carry out the immunological chemotherapy (immunity + chemotherapy) or immunological chemotherapy radiotherapy (immunity + radiotherapy) so as to reform the unilateral therapeutic outlook of singly killing the cancer cells into an all-round therapeutic outlook of killing the cancer cells as well as improving the immunity of the organism.

How to do well in assistant chemotherapy after operation? It is held by us that attention shall be paid to the following:

1. As to the patients receiving the radical operation on the cancerous protuberance, the fresh tumor specimen shall be selected for the chemotherapy drug sensitive test so as to individualize the assistant chemotherapy after operation to avoid the blindness of drug administration.

2. How to judge or estimate whether the remnant cancer cells exist in the body after radical operation so as to determine the indication of the assistant chemotherapy after operation, in this way, the immunity indexes and the tumor signs shall be detected.

3. How to judge the curative effect of the assistant chemotherapy after operation? Are the cancer cells killed or not? Since the tumor is removed, the curative effect cannot be judged as per the existence of the tumor of the volume of the tumor. The immunity indexes, the cytokines and the tumor signs shall be detected to judge the possibility of the reoccurrence and metastasis after operation.

4. **The drug administered for the assistant chemotherapy after operation shall differ from the one for primary tumor or the metastasis cancer lesion because the goals are different: the former is to eliminate the primary cancer lesion and the latter is to eliminate the residual cancer cells, as a result, the dosage shall be different and it shall be greatly reduced.**

5. The patient receiving the radical operation on cancer is very weak in the body condition and inferior in immunologic function, so the assistant chemotherapy after operation must be accompanied with the immunological mediation and control therapy, namely the immunological therapy + chemotherapy, called immunological chemotherapy. As above-mentioned, **the elimination of the cancer cells in metastasis or the cancer cells**

or the cancer cell group in the blood circulation after operation mainly depends on the immunological cells in the organism of the host. It is shown by the experimental study that the immunological cells in the organism **can eliminate 10⁵ cancer** cells, so the dosage for the assistant chemotheray after operation shall not be too large under the precondition of not damaging or slihgtly damaging the immunological cells because it is very important to carry out the immunological mediation and control therapy and improve the immunity of the organism to eliminate the cancer cells in metastasis. We deeply realize that in the past 16 years, Wuhan Shuguang Tumor Special Clinic under Wuhan Research Institute of Anti-cancerometastasis and Anti-reoccurrence has diagnosed so many patients like this, some of them are of valetudinarianism or accompanied with other diseases, resulting in failure to chemotherapy and radiotherapy; some of them fail to the chemotherapy again due to the severe response after 1-2 chemotherapy after operation; some of them refuse the chemotherapy after operation; most of the patients meet with the cancer invading serosa and are accompanied by metastasis of lymph node, so they take XZ-C medicine for treatment in the new mode of XU ZE new concept of anti-cancerometastasis treatment and orally take XZ-C medicine for a long term, resulting in a relatively good curative effect.

6. Although the assistant chemotherapy after operation has been widely popularized all over the country at present, there are short of the forward-looking, comparable and appreciable reports on the assistant chemotherapy after operation. According to the report on 5-year's follow-up survey of the assistant chemotherapy or radiotherapy after operation on the patients suffering from the stomach cancer by American Stomach Cancer Group, it was reported by Lence (1994, 3, 3, 1390) that the total survival rate was still low in the patients suffering from the stomach cancer even the patients with the cancer removed through operation, therefore, the people hope to improve the prognosis through the assistant chemotherapy and radiotherapy for the patients with low tumor load after operation. It was shown by the results of the assistant treatment with mitomycin and fluorouracil on the first group of the patients in 1976 by British Stomach Cancer Organization that it had no benefit to the patients after operation, for this reason, the study on the assistant treatment of another group of patients had been made.

The forward-looking, random and contrapositive grouping study had been made on 430 patients suffering from the gastric gland cancer in Stage II and III after operation, accompanied with radiotherapy or the combined chemotherapy of mitomycin, adriamycin and fluorouracil (MAF) plan over 5 years, among which 372 patients died, 7 of which died of the surgical complication and 327 of which died of the reoccurrence of tumor. In the random grouping study, 145 cases only adopted the operation therapy; 153 cases accepted the assistant chemotherapy with the rang of irradiation including hilum of spleen and porta hepatic with the dosage of 4500cGy and the increase in dosage of 500cGy in operative field area; another 138 cases accepted the combined chemotherapy (MPA Plan) with mitomycin 4mg/m², adriamycin 30mg/m² and fluorouracil 600 mg/m², intravenously injected, 3 weeks as a cycle, totaling 6 cycles. The total two-year's survival rate of this group of patients was 33% and the total five-year's survival rate was

17% (13%~21%), compared with the patients with the single operation therapy, as to the patients accepting the assistant chemotherapy, the survival rate was not raised: the five-year's survival rate of the patients with single operation therapy was 20% and the one of the patients accepting the operation plus radiotherapy was 19%.

Therefore, operation is still the standard therapeutic method of the stomach cancer and the assistant therapeutic measures shall be restricted within a certain scope of study.

To sum up, it is held by the author: some large hospitals or medical centers in China should make the forward-looking comparable grouping study to obtain a large number of appreciable scientific data in China. At present, the assistant chemotherapy after operation is still restricted within a certain scope of study.

This topic is in my monograph "new concept and new way of cancer treatment ". In this book in the international community it is the first time to initiative that cancer surgery after rejuvenation chemotherapy should be reformed and innovated:

This initiative will cause the work of the General Surgery and Chemotherapy Division of China's top three hospitals to the preparation of redeployment, to **change the postoperative adjuvant chemotherapy to perioperative adjuvant chemotherapy, the postoperative chemotherapy is the implementation of the surgeon and surgical nurses, that is, the surgeon and surgery nurses conduct the postoperative treatment and follow-up, so** that the statistical results of the recent short-term efficacy and long-term efficacy can be understood ; because the surgeon understands the patient's condition, the surgeon should determine whether the need for chemotherapy and chemotherapy or not? This is suitable for the actual condition, improve efficacy. However, chemotherapy department can greatly reduce the work of the preparation. This will be a major improvement measures to improve the quality of medical care and improve the level of team therapy. (See Chapter 17 P119)

6

The opinion of improvement and perfection of the traditional chemotherapy cancer treatment

- *Discussion about the "get" and "lost" after the use of anti-cancer drugs*
- *The status of tumor chemotherapy is the main reason for further improvement of efficacy*
- *Suggestions for improving and improving chemotherapy*

I.   On "gain" and "loss" after taking anti-cancer drugs

The treatment of cancer, no matter in early stage, mid stage or advanced stage, involves the comprehensive multi-discipline treatment.

The operation is a method of local treatment. The surgical oncology scientists hold that the cancer occurs locally at first, then encroaches the peripheral tissues and transfers to other places via lymphatic vessel and blood vessel, as a result, they stress on the local treatment, that is to say, the stress on control over the local growth and diffusion, especially when the cancer meets with metastasis via lymph, the lymph node is cleaned down by operation. For years, although the operative treatment has been improved continually in methodology, the long-term curative effects have not made remarkable progress as yet. The reoccurrence and metastasis after operation seriously threatens the prognosis of the patients, attracting high attention from the medical field, however, there has been no effective prescription up to now.

The radiotherapy is also a method of local treatment, which plays a role in killing off the cells from the local tumor per unit dosage. The radiotherapy effects are mostly affected by the factors including oxygenation of cells, type of tumor and restoration of cells and so on, all these characteristics determine that the radiotherapy is locally inferior to the surgical removal with respect to tumor.

The biological characteristics of cancer are invasion, reoccurrence and metastasis, which are the important reasons why the treatment with operation and radiotherapy fails.

In recent years, some one holds that cancer is a kind of generalized disease, so the generalized treatment should mainly depend on radiotherapy, however, it is a pity, in despite of the emerging new drugs and continually undated therapeutic methods and plans, the radiotherapy effects are not satisfactory. Since the cytotoxic drugs have no selectivity, they kill the cancer cells as well as the normal cells of the host, especially the immunological cells, in addition, they have severe side effects, inhibiting hematopiesis function of the bone marrow and reducing the immunity. Therefore, the traditional radiotherapy does not entirely conform to the well-known actual conditions of the biological behaviors of the cancer at present, for example, the invasion behaviors and metastasis of the cancer cells are of multi-link and multi-step. At present, people have cognized that the anti-tumor drugs do not always prevent the metastasis and reoccurrence.

In 1980s, the tumorous bioremediation emerged, such as immunological therapy, cytokine therapy and gene vaccination therapy. It was proven that some therapies could mediate the immunity of the patients, however, it has not proven that which immunological preparation or method could induce the extinction of tumor.

In the recent 20 years, so many reports on treatment of cancer with traditional Chinese medicine have been made and its outlook has been concerned by the people. Especially, with the further development of the study on medicine and immunology, people have realized that the disorder of the immune system of the organism is closely related to the occurrence and development of tumor and traditional Chinese medicine has its own characteristics and advantages in tumor treatment through mediating the immunologic function of the organism. The immunoregulation of traditional Chinese medicine and development of immunoregulator of traditional Chinese medicine will attract more attention and favor all over the world. With the assistance of operation, radiotherapy and chemotherapy, the traditional Chinese medicine can bring its immunoregulation into full play in the process of treatment and obviously prolong the survival time and improve the survival quality, in this way, the characteristics and advantages of the traditional Chinese medicine are fully embodied, however, it is disadvantageous in unremarkably improving the tumor.

Since the above-mentioned methods have different characteristics in action mechanism and effect with respect to treatment of cancer and different curative effects as well as their own disadvantages, so it is necessary to focus on the advantages and disadvantages of various therapies aiming at the "gain" and the "loss" of the paints, for example, what's the "advantage" and the "disadvantage" after taking the therapy, what's the "gain" and the "loss" of the patients? We should learn from the strong points of one therapy to offset the weakness of the other therapies and combine these therapies organically and reasonably to form the comprehensive therapeutic plans for cancer, only in this way, can the side effects from the drugs be obviously reduced, the survival quality of the patients be improved and the total survival time be prolonged. In the past 16 years, Tumor Specialized Clinic of Shuguang Tumor Research Institute has treated over 12000 cancer patients in mid and advanced stage with XZ-C immunoregulation therapy in practice and most of the patients have achieved the effects of improving the survival quality, stabilizing the lesion, controlling the metastasis, keeping survival with tumor and remarkably prolonging the survival time.

II. **Actual conditions of chemotherapy in tumor: main cause affecting further improvement of curative effects of chemotherapy**

The total effective rate of treatment with anti-tumor drug in clinic is only 14%, the factors impeding chemotherapy' better curative effects mainly include:

1. **Blindness of current chemotherapy**. Now it is unknown whether the chemical medicine used in the current therapeutic plan for chemotherapy is sensitive to the cancer cells of the patients just because most of the patients are not subject to the drugsensitive test to cancer cells. If the medicine is used by experience, it has blindness, that is to say, it may be beneficial to some patients while harmful to other patients. Based on the drugsensitive test results, remarkable curative effects have been made in treating the infectious diseases with antibiotics, as enlightens us on reasonably and jointly administrating drug through testing the sensitivity of the cancer cells of the patients to the cytotoxic drugs for chemotherapy so as to replace the blind chemotherapy with "individualized" chemotherapy. It is shown by the data that it can double the effective rate of chemotherapy.

2. **Drug resistance of chemotherapy**. Most of the solid tumor, such as stomach cancer, cancer of large intestine, is lowly sensitive or insensitive to the chemotherapy. Some tumor is remitted after chemotherapy, however, it meets with reoccurrence, resulting in ineffective chemotherapy, indicating that the cancer cells has the drug resistance to the chemotherapy drug. The reasons why the drug resistance appears include many factors such as drug transmission disturbance of solid tumor, cell proliferation, difference in dynamics, immunity and metabolism and so on.

3. Selectivity toxicity of chemotherapy anti-cancer drug. The chemotherapy drug is the cytotoxic drug, killing the cancer cells as well as the normal histiocytes, without selectivity, especially the hemopoietic stem cells of the bone marrow with exuberant proliferation and immunological cells as well as stomach cells and intestinal cells. Compared with the volume of the normal tissue, since the cancerous protuberance only accounts for a minimal proportion, it is possible to "kill one hundred enemies while injuring three thousand soldiers on one's own side". The blindness of chemotherapy and the drug resistance of chemotherapy result in low curative effects, in case that it is expected to improve the curative effects by means of increasing the dosage, increasing the kinds of drugs and shortening the time, the toxic effects will be further aggravated, so the chemotherapy in cancer is still satisfactory in despite of great progress. The drugs shall be selected by testing the sensitivity and drug resistance of the chemotherapy drug so as to have a definite object in view. If the drugsensitive test is made on the chemotherapy patients so as to avoid the damage on the patients from the blind chemotherapy and benefit the chemotherapy patients, the epoch of chemotherapy will be opened up.

III. Suggestion on improving and perfecting the chemotherapy in cancer

Since nitrogen mustard drugs were reported by Gillman and Phillips in 1946 to treat the tumor in hematopiesis function, the chemotherapy has made great progress for 60 years and the great achievements have been made in therapeutics of the malignant tumor, for example, the chemotherapy has cured over 10 kinds of malignant tumor including chorionepithilioma, acute lymphocytic leukemia, Hodgkin disease, seminoma of testis, small-cell carcinoma of the lung and Wilms tumor and so on, and remitted the tumor including breast cancer, children' lymphadenoma, neuroblastoma and osteosarcoman and so on, resulting in prolonged survival time. Thus three principles of treatment including operation, chemotherapy and radiotherapy are established. Since the chemotherapy has made great achievements, especially in the recent 20 years, it has been widely used for various solid tumor, especially in the assistant treatment after operation, so the metastasis and dissemination in some patients has been restrained and improved, giving hope to treatment of solid tumor after operation. However, it is a pity that the reoccurrence and the metastasis happen again after several months and the patients still die of the cancer despite chemotherapy or intensive chemotherapy again. According to the follow-up survey to over 12000 metastasis and reoccurrence patients and the analysis of and experience in treatment summarization in Tumor Specialized Clinic of Shuguang Tumor Research Institute, it is found neither metastasis nor the reoccurrence could not be restrained on thousands of patients receiving the assistant chemotherapy after operation, the survival time and the survival time without cancer are not obviously improved. At present, although the assistant chemotherapy after operation has been made all over the country, there has been no prospective and correlatable scientific data, the assistant chemotherapy after operation is still in study. Of course, there are lots of patients receiving assistant chemotherapy after operation who have been in good condition over 10 years even 20 years, however, due to lack of prospective and correlatable scientific data, what is the comparison result between chemotherapy and non-chemotherapy in the patients after operation? What is the long-term survival rate of the patients not subject to chemotherapy? How to prove the long-term survival results from the chemotherapy after operation? All of these issues shall be further studied. At present, the reports in China lack lots of prospective and correlatable follow-up survey analysis data as well as the prospective and correlatable evaluation data about the assistant chemotherapy after operation just because the case history is kept by the patient instead of the hospital, as a result, the doctors and the hospital cannot make the follow-up survey. Of course, the in-hospital case history is kept for study, however, the in-hospital case history just reflects the short-term curative effects, most of the effects reflected in the in-hospital case history are relatively good because if it is not so good, the patient is not allowed to leave hospital. However, most patients are in good condition temporarily, for example, after the incision heals up, the patient begins to take food again and takes case of itself, the short-term curative effects are good, but it is hardly realized that the cancer cells may be in metastasis and it cannot be tested at present, of course, some tumor markers can be dynamically observed, such as CEA and AFP and so on.

Then, how to make the further study? Start from the existing problems to settle the problems through experiments and clinical study. The treatment of cancer shall be people-oriented and aim at curing the sickness to save the patient.

1. **Actively searching, studying and developing intelligent anti-cancer drugs.** The main contradictions in chemotherapy have been mentioned above and now we should pay attention to how to study and perfect them. The main issue is: the chemotherapy is the cytotoxic drug, without selectivity, so it cannot selectively distinguish the cancer cells from the normal cells, killing off all of them, resulting in some side effects and contradictions. So we should update the thought and actively study, search and develop the "intelligent anti-cancer drug" that only selectively kills the cancer cells instead of

the normal cells of the organism, especially the immunological cells. In June 2004, American Society of Clinical Oncology held the annual meeting in New Orleans, with over 20000 oncologists as the attendants and 3700 papers called. Among these 3700 papers, there were 30 papers greatly affecting the treatment of cancer, of which there were 9 papers discussing the intelligent anti-cancer drugs. The intelligent anti-cancer drugs only affect the specific molecules in the cancer cells. The research findings of intelligent anti-drugs come into the world, indicating the treatment of cancer would shift to the epoch of accurate administration with little side effects from the one of chemotherapy with very great side effects. In research and development of the intelligent anti-cancer drugs, the research and development personnel do not spread these drugs at present. I believe that in the coming future, with the wide use of these drugs, people would feel the great effects from them and the patients would benefit from them. **Among the 48 kinds of anti-cancer drugs with relatively good tumor-inhibiting rate screened by this lab from 200 kinds of natural vegetable drugs, there are 3 kinds of vegetable drugs that can entirely inhibit and kill the cancer cells entirely and has no effects on the cultured epithelial cells or fibrous cells in the culture in vitro experiment on cancer cells, including XZ-C1-A, XZ-C1-B and XZ-C1-C. In the in vivo tumor-inhibition experiment on tumor-bearing animals, their tumor-inhibiting rate is 85%-95%. They are a part of XZ-C1, XZ-C immunoregulation anti-cancer medicine.** This experiment takes chemotherapy drug CTX as the control group and CTX obviously inhibits the immunity and the bone marrow. XZ-C anti-cancer medicine has no effects on bone marrow.

2. **Suggestion on immunologic chemotherapy.** Namely immunological treatment + chemotherapy. The immunological drugs can be administered in peri-chemotherapy period so as to reduce the side effects from chemotherapy; after chemotherapy, the immunologic treatment should be continued for a period to enhance the curative effects. The immunological treatment is the most reasonable treatment, it is of 0 order kinetics, however, it ① has relatively small acting force, it acts on 10^{5-6} cancer cells strongly; beyond this range, it acts weakly. ②The immunological drug can improve the immunity of the organism and enhance the immunological surveillance in the organism. ③ It can be continually administered or taken orally. Because the cancer cells are continually divided and proliferated, the treatment shall be also continual. XZ-C immunoregulation medicine can protect the hematopiesis function of the bone marrow, protect the thymus, improve the immunity, improve the symptom and raise the life quality; the action is relatively slowly, little but durably. Since the biological characteristics of the cancer cells are the continual division and proliferation, our countermeasures must be also continual.

Chemotherapy and immunological treatment currently adopted should learn from other's strong points to offset one's weakness and be comprehensively applied so as to improve the curative effects. The chemotherapy is of intermittent administration while the immunoregulation treatment is of continual treatment. If both of them assist with each other, the curative effects will be improved undoubtedly. If the cancer patient has inferior immunologic function, the operation on cancer will bring down the immunologic function further. In operation, the cancer cells entering the blood circulation by extrusion increase. How to eliminate or control the cancer cells entering the blood circulation in operation? It is held by us that XZ-C medicine should be added before, in and after operation for immunological treatment. $XZ-C_4$ can protect the thymus and $XZ=C_8$ can protect the bone marrow. In this way, the central immune organ and immunologic function of the host can be protected, the curative effects of the chemotherapy can be strengthened and the side effects of the chemotherapy inhibiting the immunologic function can be reduced, as a result, it will reduce the opportunity of metastasis of cancer cells, therefore, the improvement of immunologic function of the patient in the peri-operation period or in the period of assistant chemotherapy after operation is an important link of comprehensive treatment.

3. **Making sensitivity test of chemotherapy drugs and implementing "individualized" immunological chemotherapy.** Now the chemotherapy in cancer has stepped into the stage of "individualized" chemotherapy in many hospitals. Previously, the different cancer patients are subject to the same chemotherapy plan, unavoidably resulting in blindness, not conforming to the actual conditions of the patients. It is shown by the study that even though the same kind of tumor with same type of tissue, even the different stages of the same cancer, has different sensitivities to the chemotherapy drugs, therefore, it is necessary to make the drugsensitive test on the individual cancer patients and it is urgent to select the sensitive drugs from various anti-cancer drugs. It is proven by the clinical experience in chemotherapy that the effective rate of administration by experience is very low (14%), if the drug can be selected according to the results measured by drugsensitive test, the effective rate can be raised to 28%-35%.

The effect of chemotherapy in the solid tumor is not as good as the one in malignant tumor in the blood system and the transmission hindrance of drug in the solid tumor is the upmost factor of drug resistance of solid tumor.

It is an important way and one of the current study hotspots to make the sensitive test on chemotherapy drug for tumor and carry out the individualized chemotherapy plan so as to improve the effects of chemotherapy in tumor and reduce the side effects.

Generally, the drugsensitive test on tumor can be made with the method of culture in vitro and culture in vivo, the former includes cell culture method and tissue culture method and the latter refers to the method of culture in vivo in animal. Among the test methods, the method of transplantation in vivo in the nude mice can obtain true and reliable results with respect to drug test or new drug screening, however, the process is long, the operation is complicated and the price is high. The method of cell culture is the most simple, convenient and feasible, however, since the kinetics is not entirely same to the tumor in vivo, the test results often differ from the drug reaction of the tumor in vivo, so it cannot be used to directly guide the administration of the different tumor patients.

Someone makes a study on 3D tissue culture method of tumor, namely Hoffman 3D tissue culture method, which directly uses the clinical samples, avoids the repeated digestion of tumor cells with enzyme or mechanically and features quickness and relatively high success ratio. This method would be helpful to guide the individualized chemotherapy, improve the chemotherapy effects and reduce the drug resistance.

(1)   In vitro drugsensitive test: it is very important to establish the reliable anti-cancer in vitro drugsensitive test method so as to help the clinicians select the effective chemotherapy drugs, reasonably design the therapeutic method, improve the curative effects, avoid the side effects from the ineffective drugs and directly screen the new anti-cancer and anti-metastasis drugs with the fresh human tumor samples.

There are so many methods of in vitro sensitive test of anti-cancer drug and they have the common characteristics: simple method, high sensitivity, smaller dose than the in vivo method, quick judgment results, without too many animals; in addition, they also can screen the anti-cancer drugs and most of them are parallel to the in vivo method with respect to the procedures.

(2)   in vivo chemotherapy drug sensitive test: at present, as to the chemotherapy drug sensitive test methods, the in vitro method prevails and it has the advantages of quickness, convenience and simple as well as good clinical correlation and good repeatability, however, it also has some disadvantages because it breaks away from the in vivo environment of the tumor and is not consistent with the human tumor in histology and cell kinetics, reducing the coincidence rate of the test results and the clinic.

Various drugs have different concentrations in the body fluid and are affected by the body weight, route of medication, liver and kidney function and so on, in this way, the in vitro method cannot represent the change in drug concentration. Some drugs should be activated and metabolized in vivo before playing a role in anti-cancer, such as CTX; some drugs acting on the cancer cells will bring into play through the immune system. The reaction of the cancer cells to these drugs cannot be tested with in vitro method.

The solid tumor are the spatial structure occupying a certain space. Besides the tumor cells in blood, breast and ascites are directly contact with the drugs, the solid tumor is not so simple. The drugs cannot reach up to the deep part easily; the anoxia caused by ischemia; the uneven blood flow in the tumor; the difference in PH value and osmotic pressure will affect the sensitivity of the solid tumor cells to the chemotherapy drugs.

It is necessary to select the optimal "individualized" joint chemotherapy plan through the drugsensitive test.

7

the basic model and specific programs of anti-cancer metastasis

- *The basic pattern of anti-cancer metastasis*
- *The specific treatment plansof anti-cancer metastasis*
- *Immunotherapy plays an important role in anticancer treatment*

Traditional chemotherapy against metastasis mainly aims to kill cancer cells. No matter it is the primary carcinoma, metastatic carcinoma, the postoperative adjuvant chemotherapy preventing reoccurrence and metastasis or when metastasis of lymph nodes is found, intravenous chemotherapy drugs are adopted in all cases. However, because chemotherapy drugs are of no selectivity and kill both cancer cells and normal cells (especially the immunological cells), they act as a double-edged sword. The author holds that various schemes for intravenous chemotherapy are mainly the different combinations of cytotoxic drugs, which are not certainly in line with the multi-link and multi-step biological characteristics of the cancerometastasis process.

I. The basic model of anti-cancerometastasis treatment

Among the innumerable patients in this clinical practice, it is not uncommon to see that some of them are not free from metastasis after the postoperative adjuvant chemotherapy. What is worse is that some of them suffered a simultaneous metastasis in chemotherapy or suffered from the metastasis again after chemotherapy again. All these phenomena make us deeply think about the reason behind the failure to prevent metastasis. Is it the traditional chemotherapy not in line with the biological characteristics of cancerometastasis process? Whether it is necessary to update our knowledge and thinking, or to change our conceptions and treatment model on anti-canceromestasis? Xu Ze's design concept of anti-cancerometastasis countermeasures is just an innovation of the concepts, thinking, methods and models of the traditional anti-metastasis treatment.

Anti-metastasis drugs tend to interfere or blockade a certain link or step of the metastasis process of cancer cells or the cancer cell clusters so as to inhibit the formation of metastasis focus. Although the chemotherapeutic cytotoxic drugs can kill tumor cells, suspend the growth of primary carcinoma and delay the occurrence time of metastasis, they fail to inhibit the process of invasion and metastasis. At present, the ideal drugs killing the primary carcinoma and inhibiting invasion and metastasis are unavailable. Thus, it is necessary to study the strategy of interdiction, prevention and treatment aiming at the development steps and mechanism of the cancerometastasis summarized as "eight steps and three stages".

The invasion and metastasis of carcinoma is a complicated process of many steps and the metastasis process could be generalized as following: proliferation of primary cancerous protuberance→ the formation and growth of newly born micrangium of tumor→ invading and breaking through basement membrane→ cancer cells breaking away from parent tumor and breaking through basement membrane and then perforating micrangiums or micro lymphatic vessels→ the survival and floating of invading blood in the circulatory system→ formation of small cancer embolus from cancer cells clusters wrapped by blood platelet and delivery to remote target organs together with blood stream→ the detention in the micrangium of target organs→ the attachment or adherence of cancer embolus to the wall of micrangium→ breaking through blood vessels and forming micro metastasis focus→formation of newly born micrangium of tumor as the metastasis focus→ the proliferation of the metastasis focus. If we could find the way to blockade one or several links or steps, it is possible to control metastasis, as is the context in which Xu Ze's new model of anti-cancerometastasis treatment is formed and developed.

II. **The specific plan of anti-cancerometastasis treatment**

According to biological behaviors of modern oncology on cancerometastasis and theory of reoccurrence and metastasis, this libratory has been always searching for new anti-metastasis drugs among traditional Chinese herbs extracted from natural herbs for years. Through experimental study on of tumor-bearing animal bodies with traditional Chinese medicine as well as the combination of traditional Chinese medicine and western medicine, we interfere, obstruct and intercept all the links of the metastasis, and develop an anti-metastasis scheme and countermeasure with XZ-C medicine, including XZ-C-TG against the formation of micrangium, XZ-C-AS dissolving cancer embolus, XZ-C-MD against invading into and breaking through blood vessels, XZ-C-LM with antigenicity, XZ-C-Ind against PGE2; VA and XZ-C-CA as calcium channel blocking drugs against invasion, XZ-C-GB against adherence, XZ-C-TIMP against the resistance to drugs, $XZ-C_1$ inhibiting cancer cells rather than normal cells; $XZ-C_4$ protecting thymus and improving immunity; $XZ-C_8$ protecting bone marrow and improving hematogenesis function and Emulsion of Brucea Javanica into lymph nodes. The comprehensive measures of the above-mentioned treatment schemes have achieved sound curative effects in the clinical practice by our anti-cancer cooperative group.

Because cancerometastasis is a complicated process of multi-step and multi-link, it is necessary to adopt the comprehensive measures in an all-round way to treat the cancerometastasis instead of a certain drug or measure. Thus aiming at the steps of metastasis, we scientifically design and adopt different treatment schemes and countermeasures shown in the following table. Those treatment schemes and countermeasures aiming at the steps of metastasis are to achieve the same goal of anti-metastasis.

Authors: Xu Ze (China) ; Xu Jie(China) ; Bin Wu(America)

The new model of anti-cancerometastasis treatment of Xu Ze's new concept (treatment schemes and countermeasures for the steps of canceromestasis)

Metastasis step	Treatment countermeasures	XZ-C medicine and its role
Proliferation of primary cancerous	Operation, chemotherapy	$XZ-C_1$ inhibiting cancer cells $XZ-C_4$ protecting thymus and improving immunity $XZ-C_8$ protecting bone marrow and improving hematogenesis function
Growth of newly born micrangium of tumor	Inhibiting the formation of micrangium	XZ-C-TG against formation of micrangium XZ-C-CA against adherence
Invasion into basement membrance	Anti-adhesion, anti-kinesalgia and inhibiting the activity of hydrolase	XZ-C-K(LWF) against adhesion Ind against PGE2 XZ-C-MD against kinesalgia
Breaking through blood vessels or lymphatic vessels	Anti-adhesion, anti-kinesalgia and inhibiting the activity of hydrolase	XZ-C-MD against invasion into blood vessels XZ-C-K (LWF) $XZ-C_{1+4}$ mediating immunity
In the blood of circulatory system	Inhibiting the aggregation and coagulation of blood platelet. Biological response modification (BRM)	XZ-C-N (CZR) against the aggregation of blood platelet XZ-C-LM XZ-C-ASP dissolving cancer embolus $XZ-C_{1+4}$ mediating immunity
The formation of cancer embolus	Promoting blood circulation and removing stasis and resisting thrombus	XZ-C-K (NSR) against cancer embolus XZ-C-N (CZR) against aggregation of blood platelet
The breaking out of cancer embolus from blood vessels	Resisting adhesion, kinesalgia, and the activity of hydrolase	XZ-C-MD against the breaking out of cancer embolus
The formation of metastasis focus	Operation, radiotherapy, chemotherapy	$XZ-C_{1+4}$ mediating immunity XZ-C-TG inhibiting the growth of blood vessels
The metastasis of lymph nodes	Liposoluble drugs	The Emulsion of Brucea Javanica as the carrier of lipa entering into the lymph nodes

The correlative factors of the invasion of cancer cells are adherence, enzymatic secretion and kinesalgia. The inhibition of adhesion, kinesalgia and enzymatic secretion is also helpful to inhibit the exfoliation of cancer cells from parent tumor, its break into matrix and the formation of the newly born blood vessels of the tumor besides its contribution to prevent the invasion of primary carcinoma. For years the researches on inhibitors inhibiting the growth of newly born blood vessels are seen in reports. Meanwhile, it is also discovered in the tumor-bearing animal experiment screening the anti-cancerometastasis drugs by this libratory that traditional Chinese medicine TG is of sound inhibiting effects on newly born blood vessels. Tumor cells are in weakest condition to resist the host environment when entering into the blood of the circulatory system and can be easily eliminated by the immunological cells of the host. It is proved by some literature that a vast majority of cancer cells entering into the circulatory system are killed by immunological cells and only a number of approximately 0.01% thereof could survive and possibly become the focus of metastasis. Except the mechanical damage factors, the cancer cells in blood stream are mainly eliminated by the damaging effects of the immunological function of the hosts against tumor cells. Tumor-bearing patients usually suffer low immunological function inhibited by tumor and chemotherapy. Therefore, it is necessary to adopt immunotherapy, biotherapy and biological response modification and traditional Chinese medicine for immunological mediation to protect the function of immune organs so as to improve the immunity of the host. It is found that XZ-C medicine can protect bone marrow and improve hemogenesis function, protect hemogenesis function of bone marrow as well as stem cells, improve immunologic function and inhibit the metastasis of tumor. According to the clinical application on the innumerable patients in the clinic of Anti-cancer Cooperative Group of Traditional Chinese Medicine Combined with Western Medicine over ten years, XZ-C medicine against cancer and metastasis has achieved significant curative effects.

III. **The important role of immunotherapy in anti-cancerometastasis treatment**

Among all the current therapeutic methods, operation and radiotherapy are both local therapy while chemotherapy, immunotherapy, biological therapy, therapy with traditional Chinese medicine are systematic therapy. At present, the chemotherapy mainly targets the focus of primary cancer or metastasis focus and the criterion to judge the curative effects is to alleviate and shrink the tumor. In order to fulfill of the above criterion, a significant dose of chemotherapeutic cytotoxic drugs are in need to shrink the lump. Additionally in view of the cell cycle, medicines are necessarily combined in order to achieve a certain level of lethality. If it is a $1cm \times 1cm^2$ lump, it would contain a number of 10^{12} cancer cells and this, requires a considerable dose of chemotherapeutic drugs to shrink it into half. However, it only needs a slight dose if cancer cells are eliminated in the process of metastasis by chemotherapy, because the amount of cancer cells in metastasis process only accounts to 10^7 to 10^8 and most of them could be eliminated. The problem happens as a large amount of immunological cells in blood circulation are destroyed by chemotherapeutic cytotoxic drugs whereas the anti-metastasis mainly depends on the system against cancer cells of the organism itself. Thus it would be a great loss to patients. Chemotherapy could only be conducted with intermission during which time a large amount of cancer cells and immunological cells would be both eliminated. However there still exist a handful of escaped cancer cells during this period which continually split and proliferate or are even more active. <u>More than that, the destroyed immunological cells, decreased immunity and weakened immune surveillance would also lead or contribute to the development and metastasis of cancer cells.</u>

Therefore, the chemotherapeutic drugs should not be overdosed in the anti-metastasis treatment and should not impair a large amount of immunological cells. Meanwhile, chemotherapy should be accompanied by Immunotherapy, Biotherapy, Biological Response Modification (BRM), XZ-C medicine and tonic traditional Chinese medicine so as to give play to each other's advantages and make up each other's imperfections. Because a properly protected and activated immune system of the body could eliminate 10^6 cancer cells and additional chemotherapeutic drugs could destroy most cancer cells in the process of metastasis, it is possible to hold up and cut off the metastasis path and put the diffusion and metastasis under further control.

Xu Ze's new concept of anti-metastasis treatment promotes the application of immunochemotherapy, namely the combination of immunotherapy and chemotherapy. To be specific, immune drugs would be used in the peri-chemotheraputic period, in other words, at the week before the chemotherapy to be implemented, and would not be ceased in the chemotherapy period unless in case of serious chemotherapy response. The immunotherapy will continue for 6 to 9 months after chemotherapy and during intermission for the maintenance of a certain level of immunity and the consolidation of the curative effects. All these above are proved to be reasonable. For 16 years the Dawn Specialist Out-patient of our anti-metastasis laboratory uses XZ-C anti-cancer traditional Chinese medicine for immunological mediation to coordinate chemotherapy, which usually causes less chemotherapy response. Most of the postoperative in our out-patients suffer the liver, gallbladder, pancreas, stomach, intestine, lung and breast cancer. Some suffer a multi-part lymphatic metastasis after radical operations but then meet with serious response after chemotherapy thus come to our out-patient for treatment. Some fail the exploratory operation and some are under palliative operations. Therefore, the author, through combining the small-dosed chemotherapy with XZ-C medicine, usually finds less response and hemogram variation. Because of different conditions of the patients and the absence of comparability, it is impossible to conduct the comparative observation of perspective random allocation. Therefore, the perspective clinical study is conducted by comparatively observing the curative effects of the immunotherapy group and the chemotherapy group with immune indexes (IFN, IL-2 and TNF), the level of tumor marker, the quality of life and the survival time as the evaluative criteria of the two groups.

The immune drugs used in the above-mentioned immunochemotherapy shall increase the immunity indexes of the body. Actually not all traditional Chinese medicine that support healthy energy and eliminate evil are able to improve immunity because some are of **bidirectional regulating function,** which would improve immunity at a certain dosage range but lower immunity at another dosage range. For example, the glossy privet fruit could significantly increase the spleen and thymus indexes; the bupleurum roots lead to the atrophy of the mice thymus; and the liquid made from the pilose antlers of a young stag could improve the weight of the spleen and thymus of the mice if it is poured into their stomach. Additionally, barrenwort polysaccharide would lead to the atrophy of the thymus but a long-term oral administration turns to increase the weight of thymus. $XZ-C_{1+4+8}$ medicine is proved to be able to increase cytokines like IFN, IL-2, TNF etc and to decrease the level of tumor markers of many terms by many animal experiments and long-term clinical observation. To be specific, $XZ-C_4$ could protect bone marrow and thymus and improve hematopoiesis functions and immunity thus raises the overall immune level. The test by cultivating cancer cells in vitro reveals that the series of XZ-C1 medicine, including $XZ-C_1$-A, $XZ-C_1$-B and $XZ-C_1$-C, are the three pharmaceutics that 100% kill cancer cells, 100% cause no harm to normal cells and achieve an 85% to 95% tumor-inhibiting rate in tumor-inhibiting experiments on the body of tumor-bearing animals. Cyclophosphane (CTX) as the control group only achieves a tumor-inhibiting rate of 45% and also significantly decreases the immunity.

The removal of focus of primary cancer and metastasis focus depends on local surgical removal or radiation exposure. The focus of primary cancer should be removed by surgical removal if possible and in case of impossibility, it would be helpful to turn to interventional therapy, radiotherapy, radio frequency, focused ultrasound or the injection of absolute ethyl alcohol so as to control the local focus.

The metastasis of tumor is an essential expression of malignancy. The reason why cancer treatment is failed is that the treatment isn't proper and the immunity of the patients isn't sufficiently strong to kill all the cancer cells. Literatures show that a marginally small tumor (1 to 8g) could release millions or even thousand millions of cancer cells in 24 hours into blood. However, a vast majority of these cancel cells would be eliminated by the human body's immune system and only 1% of them are possibly able to survive and evolve into metastasis tumor. The test data of our libratory reveals that the immunity of mice is capable of killing 100,000 cancer cells. The amount could be increased to more than 1,000,000 if $XZ-C_1$ medicine is used. The question is what destroys them? It is the immunological cells of the body itself. Thus Xu Ze's new concept holds that the immunological cells of body should be protected and not be damaged by any treatments. It is necessary to find ways to protect and activate the immunological function of the host. It would be beneficial for the patients if the immunotherapy and a small-dosed chemotherapy are combined as immunochemotherapy, learning from each other's strong points and offsetting each other's weakness.

8

the new models and new methods of cancer treatment

- *Strengthen immunotherapy, to improve adverse reactions to chemotherapy*
- *Change intermittent treatment for continuous treatment*
- *change the damage to the host into protecting the host*
- *change the potential of the tumor and the host, and strive imbalance into the balance*
- *change from damaging the central immune organs into protecting the central immune organs*
- *change the injury therapy into non-injury therapy*

I. **Strengthening of immunological therapy and improving side effects from chemotherapy**

1. Side effects of traditional chemotherapy: when chemotherapy is made on cancer, it usually inhibits immunologic function and hematopoiesis function of the bone marrow, descends WBC and PLT and damages liver and kidney function as well as gastroenteric function, leading to the side effects such as nausea, emesis, abdominal distension, anorexia and so on.

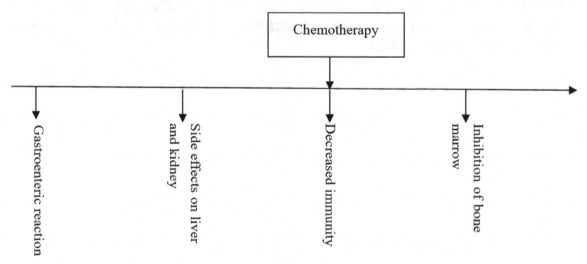

Fig. 1 Side effects of traditional chemotherapy

168

2. The countermeasures of Xu Ze's new concept: the method to improve the side effects of chemotherapy is to strengthen the supporting therapy and take effective measures to protect the host. Among the traditional Chinese medicine for immunological mediation, XZ-C$_4$ can protect thymus thus and improve immunity; XZ-C$_8$ can protect hematopoiesis function of the bone marrow and generate more stem cells; XZ-C medicine for immunity mediation can strengthen physical strength of cancerous patients. See Fig. 2.

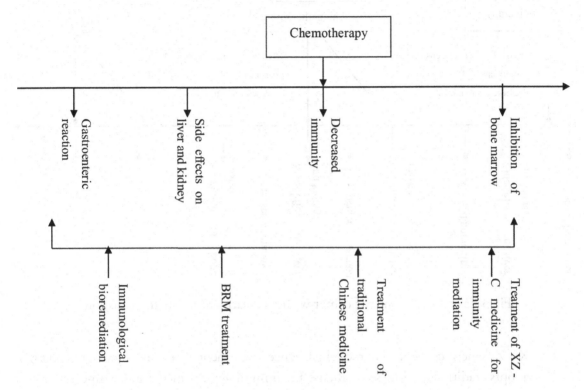

Fig. 2 Countermeasures for side effects of chemotherapy

II. Changing intermittent treatment into continual treatment

1. Traditional intravenous chemotherapy is an intermittent therapy, that is to say, after the drug for chemotherapy is applied for 3-5 days, it is necessary to apply the chemotherapeutic drug for the second course of treatment when WBC and PLT return to normal after 3-4 weeks. The drug for chemotherapy shall not be continually applied during the intermission between the first and the second course of treatment, whereas the cancel cells are still continually and uninterruptedly proliferated and divided in the intermission and increase at the speed of geometrical progression. In addition, because of the inhibition of immunologic function caused by chemotherapeutic drug, the cancel cells escape from or are free of the immunological surveillance, their proliferation and division are quickened during the intermission between these two courses, in other words, the longer the course of treatment of chemotherapeutic drug, the more the combined drug and the more the dose, the more serious of the attack against immunity

of the human body, resulting in lack of immunological surveillance, and even resulting in reoccurrence and metastasis in chemotherapy, and shrinkage of tumor firstly before continual enlargement later (see Fig. 3). These cases occur commonly, how to treat them? It is held by us that the following model should be adopted for a continuous immunological therapy in the intermission between two courses of treatment.

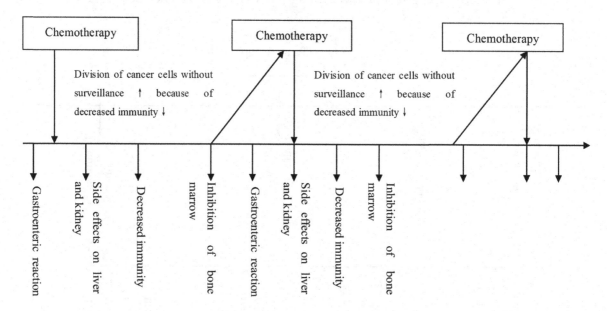

Fig.3 Easy reoccurrence of tumor without treatment in the intermission

2.   Xu Ze's new concept and model of cancer treatment is a continuous treatment. It adopts traditional Chinese medicine for immunological mediation, namely XZ-C$_1$ + XZ-C$_4$, or BRM for treatment during the intermission. XZ-C$_1$ was screened through the experimental study on tumor-bearing animals over 7 years and has been proven by a sixteen-year clinical verification that it has only inhibited the cancel cells rather than normal ones and that it can benefit spleen and stomach. XZ-C$_4$ can protect thymus from atrophy, prevent immunity from decreasing and make it better. Continual treatment in the intermittence with XZ-C medicine can control proliferation of caner cells and also protect the function of immune organs such as thymus.

The combination of chemotherapeutic drug and XZ-C medicine can decrease teh side effects from chemotherapy and strengthen chemotherapy effects against the loss of immunological surveillance as well meanwhile. See Fig. 4.

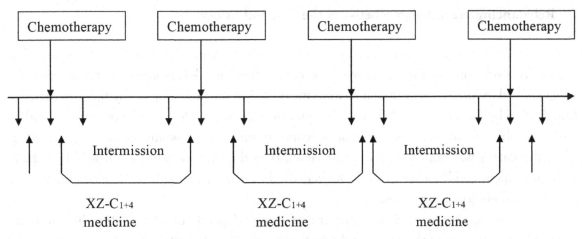

Fig. 4 Continual treatment in the intermission

III. **Therapy of protecting the host instead of damaging the host**

1. Traditional chemotherapy tends to damage the hosts: chemotherapeutic drugs are the x drugs and function as a double-edged sword, killing both cancer cells and normal ones for the lack of selectivity, inhibiting bone marrow and decreasing peripheral WBC and PLT. See Fig. 5.

2. Xu Ze' new concept and model of cancer treatment tends to protect the hosts: the new-type anticancer drugs only inhibit cancer cells, have no effects on normal cells, protect thymus, improve immunity and protect bone marrow. Among XZ-C medicine, $XZ-C_1$ only inhibits the cancel cells and have no effects on normal cells; $XZ-C_4$ protects thymus from atrophy and improves immunity; $XZ-C_8$ protects bone marrow and produces blood, all of which have been screened through the experiments on tumor-bearing animals over 7 years and have been proven by the clinical data of nearly 10000 cases in the cooperative anti-cancer clinic over 10 years. See Fig. 6.

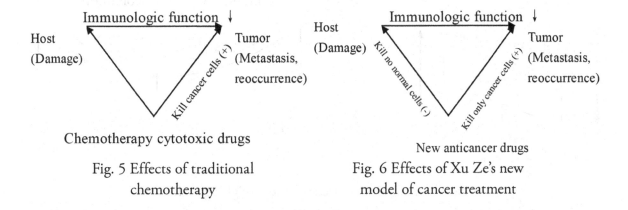

Fig. 5 Effects of traditional chemotherapy

Fig. 6 Effects of Xu Ze's new model of cancer treatment

Authors: Xu Ze (China) ; Xu Jie(China) ; Bin Wu(America)

IV. Rebalancing the unbalance between the host and tumor

It has been proven by the abovementioned findings from the experimental study that the positive relationship exists between the occurrence and development of tumor and the structure and immunologic function of immune organs of the host such as thymus and marrow. Enlightened by the seesaws in children's park and the weighing scale in the laboratory, the author took a tumble: if immunologic function was too inferior, tumor would grow up, meanwhile, when the former was improved to a certain level, then the later would be controlled in a stable or improvement condition (Fig. 7). However, the fluctuation of the level depends on further experimental observation and test.

Thus, the occurrence and development of tumor depends on the relationship between immunologic function of the host and the intrinsic biological characteristics of tumor. Similarly, the invasion and metastasis of cancer also rests with the relationship, namely, carcinoma would be put under control in case of the balance between biological characteristics of tumor cells and impacts of the host on the inhibition factors; otherwise, the cancer would grow up.

Traditional radiotherapy and chemotherapy are inclined to weakening immunologic function and lead to a worse unbalance between both of them.

Xu Ze's new model of cancer treatment aims to improve the immunity of patients as much as possible, level off the decreased *immunity* (Fig. 8) and thus inhibit tumor growth and strengthen immunological surveillance.

Immune system is the one composed of immune organs, immunological cell and molecules executing immunologic function, mainly including central lymphatic tissue, peripheral lymphatic tissue and immunological cells. Central lymphatic tissue, the home to immune cells for their occurrence, differentiation and maturation, includes thymus and bone marrow. Peripheral lymphatic tissue includes lymph nodes, spleens and stomachs, in which T cells and B cells settle and these cells make their immune response after the identification of foreign antigen.

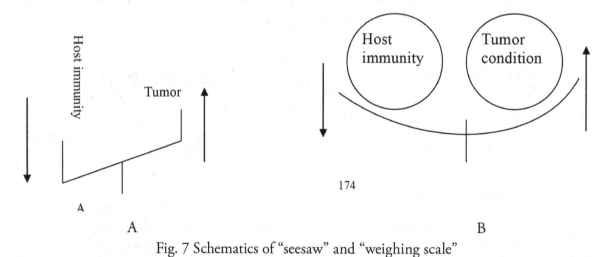

Fig. 7 Schematics of "seesaw" and "weighing scale"

A. tumor grows up in unbalance; B. stabled improvement conditions in balance

172

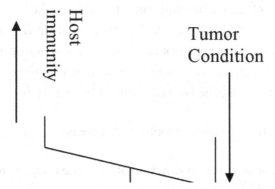

Fig. 8 Improved immunity and controlled tumor

V. Protecting central immune organs instead of damaging it

1. Traditional chemotherapy inhibits immunologic function: when cancer happens, thymus **has been inhibited by "cancer-inhibiting thymic factor**" and atrophied. Meanwhile, chemotherapy inhibits immunity and bone marrow, damages hemopoietic system and finally lead to the adynamia of the central immune organs as a whole.

    In case of cancerometastasis, a large number of cancer cells are swarming into lymph nodes and destroy their immunologic function. As to the spleen, it could inhibit or destroy cancer cells intruding in the spleen along the blood and provide nowhere for the existence of free cancer cells due to its intrinsic structures and functions. Thus there is generally no primary or secondary malignant tumor in the spleen. However, it is shown by the experiments that the immunologic function of the spleen to tumor is bidirectional, namely, it effectively inhibits tumor in the early stage of cancer but fails in the late stage.

2. Xu Ze's new model of cancer treatment can protect thymus and bone marrow and prevent the immunologic function of the host from damage. According to anatomic experiments on more than 2,000 tumor-bearing animal models, it was found that the growth of tumor is accompanied with the thymus atrophy in form of simultaneously direct proportion. In addition, the death of mice is also proportional to the tumor growth and thymus atrophy. Conclusively, it is necessary to protect thymus and improve immunity. As well as that, in studying the reason why cancer leads to death on thousands of late tumor-bearing animal models, it is found by us that the thymuses apparently atrophied among all grouped dead animals in the final stage of carcinoma, their central immune organ met with atrophy and malfunction. It may be one important reason why the cancer patients died of cancer. It is a common fact that most cancer patients die of cancer in clinic. But further careful analysis and profound consideration would reveal the close relationship between infection bleeding, the failure of organ function and adynamia of immunologic function, which enlightens us to try to prevent or inhibit

the thymus atrophy of tumor-bearing animal models in the late stage of tumor. We just aim to find the way to prevent or alleviate thymus atrophy, no matter what measure is taken. After a long-term experimental research, it is found by us that XZ-C$_4$ and XZ-C$_8$ screened from the natural herbs, the former can protect thymus and improve immunologic function and the later can protect bone marrow and produce the blood.

XZ-C$_4$ can protect thymus from atrophy and increase lymphocyte and T cells.

XZ-C$_8$ can protect hematopoiesis function of the bone marrow, rebuild erythrocyte and leucocyte system and correct anemia.

VI. Non-damage therapy instead of damage therapy

1. For half a century, the traditional anti-cancer therapies have been always the operation, the radiotherapy and the chemotherapy, the first two are the local therapy and the last one is the systematic therapy, all of which would damage the patients to a certain extent. To be specific, operations would attack the ability of the patients to resist disease at a certain level and also cause an implantation, dissemination or residue of exfoliated and free cancer cells, thus resulting in reoccurrence or metastasis after operation. Radiotherapy would cause radioactive inflammatory pathological changes. Chemotherapy has great systemic side effects on the human body. Although currently the traditional therapies have been gradually improved as regional selective local therapy with intubation or catheter on target organs, which aims to increase local concentration and narrow down the damage range of cytotoxic drug, the whole body would still under the effects of medicine disseminated systemically and be subject to obviously toxic effects such as decreased immunity, inhibition of bone marrow, gastroenteric reaction, hair shedding, renal and hepatic injuries and so on. In addition, radioactive rays and chemotherapeutic drugs are two carcinogenic factors despite of the ability of radiotherapy and chemotherapy to kill cancer cells, thus they would be obviously harmful to the patients.

2. The characteristics of the effects of the new non-damage therapy and Xu Ze's new model of cancer treatment:

Many new therapies such as biotherapy, immunotherapy, differentiation and induction therapy, gene therapy, Chinese medicine treatment, combined therapy of traditional Chinese and western medicine and so on, have been emerging in the past 10 years, most of which devote to improving immunity, protecting the host, simulating and inducing the anticancer cell clusters within the anticancer system of the host (including NK cell clusters, K cell clusters, LAK cell clusters, macrophage cell clusters and TK cell clusters) as well as the factor system of anticancer cells (including IFN, IL-2, TNF, LT), regulating and controlling neurohumor system and endocrine system, strengthening the immunologic function and antineoplastic ability of the host and maintaining a balance and sustainability for the host. Z-C medicine was screened from natural herbs on tumor-bearing experimental animals, got a remarkable curative effect by a ten-year follow-up clinical verification with data of approximate 10,000 clinical cases and categorized as non-damage medicine, which could actually constitutes a non damage therapy.

The effects of burgeoning non-damage therapy could be summarized as follows: ① directly improve the anti-tumor ability of the host; ② indirectly improve the anti-cancer ability of the host by diminishing inhibition mechanism; ③ improve the resistance power of the host against oncotherapy; ④ enhance the immunogenicity of tumors.

No matter the traditional therapy or the new concept therapy, operation is the preferred method to treat solid tumor. Radical surgery to resect tumor is the currently best therapeutic method in the range of indication. In 1960s, the author resected huge abdominal tumor more than 6kg for 4 patients, one of which was a female patient, aged 50, with a hysteroma over 18kg. Such a huge solid tumor can't be removed by chemotherapy, immunity, traditional Chinese medicine or BRM. The strategy for treatment of cancerous protuberance is to adopt different methods to eliminate the number of cancer cells to a certain order of magnitude (Someone fixes the order of magnitude at 10^6 mice cells or corresponding 3.5×10^9 human cells and describes it as a spherical nodule with a diameter of 1.5cm) and remediate the human body under this condition. Z-C$_{1+4}$ are verified by the experiments from this laboratory that they could put 10^5 cancer cells under control. Thus if XZ-C medicine is applied in adjuvant therapy after the tumors resection surgery of patients, the body resistance could be strengthened so as to eliminate pathogenic factors and diminish reoccurrence and metastasis.

9

"Three Steps" of Anti-cancer Metastasis Therapy

- *The metastasis step should be understood so that the goal of treatment is more specific*
- *Try to break each step by step*
- *Three major strategies of anti-cancer treatment (trilogy)*

[Abstract]

Objectives: Probing into the detailed strategies of therapy of carcinoma metastasis.
Methods: Deeply analyzing "Eight Steps" and "Three Stages" of carcinoma metastasis and trying to destroy the metastasis steps respectively.
Results: Putting forward the three countermeasures for therapy of carcinoma metastasis, namely "Three-Steps" through analysis.
Conclusions: The space allocation of XU ZE Three Steps of Therapy of Carcinoma Metastasis is in blood circulation and its time allocation is in three different stages. XU ZE Three Steps of Therapy of Carcinoma Metastasis attach importance to the immunity of the host and improvement of immune surveillance of the immunological cells in blood circulation on the cancer cells in the routing of metastasis.
[Keywords]: Anti carcinoma metastasis; three steps; immune surveillance

1. **The metastasis step should be understood so that the goal of treatment is more specific**

As to how to make clearer the extremely complicated dynamic and continuous biological process of carcinoma metastasis with multi-step and multi-element, through repeated thinking and carefully analysis, we summed up and put forward Eight Steps of Metastasis of Cancer Cells in the aforesaid. Based on Eight Steps, we tried to make clearer and more particular of the concept of extremely complicated dynamic and continuous biological process of carcinoma metastasis with multi-step and multi-element with respect to understanding. In order to take scientific measures to obstruct and intercept each metastasis step and destroy it one by one, it is necessary to make clear the concept of each step in the metastasis process. Only when the target of each step is made clear, can the prevention and cure countermeasures be carried out, researched and probed into.

176

In the above, we have mentioned "Three Stages" of carcinoma metastasis and illuminated it in details. The reason why "Three Stage" is put forward is that one of the keys to therapy of cancer is to anti metastasis, however, at present, the understanding of the concept of metastasis is still ambiguous and it is not clear and particular. People only understand the severity of the harm of the metastasis to the patients, however, it lacks of effective prevention and therapeutic countermeasures with clear concept and detailed profile. In order to take scientific measures to obstruct and intercept each metastasis step, based on the Eight Steps, Three Stages and the molecular mechanism of carcinoma metastasis, we try to establish the preventive and therapeutic countermeasures for each stage and called it Xu Ze Three Steps of Therapy of Carcinoma Metastasis.

2.   Try to break each step by step

The basic process of carcinoma metastasis is: the cancer cell falling from the primary tumor---degrading the basement membrance---migrating into blood capillary and small vein---survived cancer cell adhering to endothelial cell of blood capillary or basement membrane under the exposed endothelium---passing through wall---growing up in the remote target organ and forming the metastatic carcinoma, which is an extremely complicated, dynamic and continuous biological process, composed of several relatively independent but interlocked steps. In each step, a series of molecular biological events will happen between cancer cells, and between the cancer cells and the host cells, finishing the whole metastatic process and finally forming the metastatic carcinoma.

That is to say, it is necessary for the cancer cells to be subject to and finish the whole metastatic process before forming the metastatic carcinoma. any failure of each step will result in the stop of the whole metastatic process, which presents that if we take measures to destroy the metastatic steps one by one and carry out the strategy and tactics of obstruction and interception of the cancer cells in the routing of the metastasis, it is certainly possible to break or intercept the metastatic routing and intercept and kill the cancer cells in the routing of metastasis.

Xu Ze New Concept and Mode of Therapy of Carcinoma and Carcinoma Metastasis are to try to intercept one or several steps or links of the above-mentioned metastatic process so as to control the metastasis.

In order to realize the above-mentioned objectives, what measures shall be taken by us for anti metastasis? With which theory? Which technology and which drug? In which step or in which stage and link to intercept the cancer cells in the routing of the metastasis?

3.   Three Steps of Therapy of Carcinoma Metastasis or three major strategies of anti-cancer treatment (trilogy)

1.   First step of anti carcinomatous metastasis: in this stage, the metastatic process of cancer cells is as follows: cancer cells falling from the primary carcinoma---adhering to the stroma outside the cells---degrading ECM to open up a road for cancer cells---carrying out cell movement via the adherence of degraded stroma or the degraded stroma for adherence---then arriving at the external wall---degrading

basement membrane of blood vessel---doing Amoeba movement, firstly stretching out the pseudopodium---then passing through the wall.

Prevention and cure countermeasures: this stage is the intervention and repression countermeasure before the cancer cell falls from the primary carcinoma and enters the blood vessel. In this stage, the therapeutic "targets" are mainly anti-adherence, anti-degradation, anti-movement and anti cancer cell attack. The therapeutic goal is to prevent the cancer cells from entering the blood vessel so as to realize the goal of "turning the enemy back at the border".

2. Second step of anti carcinomatous metastasis: in this stage, the metastasis process of cancer cell: it will pass through the wall and enter the blood circulation. The cancer cell will be interweaved in various blood cell components including blood plasma and blood or will be adhered to cancer cell group together with homo-cancer cell, or will be adhered to slight cancer embolus together with the alloplasm such as blood platelet and white blood cell and float in venous system→turn back to the right ventricle→circulate→enter pulmonary vein→turn back to left ventricle together with the venous blood, some cancer cells can stay in the pulmonary microcirculation blood vessel (forming the pulmonary metastasis lesion), some will enter the pulmonary vein→turn back to the left ventricle via the pulmonary microcirculation. The cancer cell, interweaved in the blood, enters the aorta and then jets into the small artery of the parenchymatous viscera and then enters the microcirculation of each organ (especially the parenchymatous organ, such as liver, kidney, brain and porotic substance of bone through the impact force and vertex flow and pump flow of the heart valve blood. Most of the cancer cells in the circulation will be damaged and killed by the immunological cells in the circulation or the strong blood impact force and shearing force, the tiny minority of the survived cancer cells form the micro-cancer embolus, adhering to the endothelial cell of the micrangium, degrading the basement membrance and passing through the blood vessel.

In this stage, the cancer cell will contact various immunological cells in floating in the blood circulation and cannot survive possibly due to being captured and phagocytized by various immunological cells in the blood. Few survived cancer cells will be adhered to the endothelial cell of the blood vessel due to escaping from the monitoring of the immunity in the blood circulation.

Prevention and cure countermeasures: in this stage, the "target" of therapy of carcinoma metastasis is to protect and enhance the immunologic function of various immunological cells in the blood circulation, activate the immunological cytokine and resist adherence (homogenous adherence of cancer cells and cancer cells, alloplasmatic adherence of cancer cells with blood platelet and so on), resist movement, resist aggregation of blood platelet, resist high coagulation and resist cancer embolus.

Therapeutic goal: activating the immunological cell, protecting function of thymus organization, improving immunity, protecting the bone marrow and producing the blood and promoting the cancer cells floating in the blood circulation to be captured, phagocytized, surrounded and annihilated and intercepted by the immunological cell group.

The second step is the main battlefield to kill off the cancer cells floating in the blood circulation as well as the main countermeasures to interfere and repress the carcinoma metastasis.

3. Third Step of anti carcinomatous metastasis: the metastasis process of the cancer cell in this stage: the cancer cell escapes the monitoring of the immunological cell in blood circulation and the annihilation of the immunological cell, passes through the wall and anchors itself in the organs with agreeable local microenvironment for settlement, in this way, the new blood capillary of tumor forms and then it gradually forms the metastatic carcinoma.

Prevention and cure countermeasures: the interference and repression countermeasures, mainly aiming at improving the histogenic immunity of the local microenvironment and regulating the local microenvironment to make it adverse to the survival and nidation and repress the angiogenesis factor and the new angiogenesis.

To sum up, space allocation of Xu Ze Three Steps of Therapy of Carcinoma Metastasis is in the blood circulation and the time allocation is in three different stages. It attaches importance to improvement of the host immunity. It can be summed up and concluded as Table 1

Table 1 Xu Ze Three Steps of Therapy of Carcinoma Metastasis

Metastasis stage of cancer cell	Metastasis process	Prevention and cure countermeasures
The stage before the cancer cell intrudes the circulation First step of anti metastasis	Separating the cancer cell from the primary cancer→degrading ECM→adherence and de-adherence→movement→before entering the blood vessel.	• anti-adherence • anti-degradation • anti-movement • anti stroma metal protease

Authors: Xu Ze (China) ; Xu Jie(China) ; Bin Wu(America)

Transportation stage of cancer cell in blood circulation
Second step of anti-metastasis

The cancer cell group and micro cancer embolus float in the blood circulation and are damaged due to being phagocytized and captured by the immunological cell and be subject to the shearing force of the blood.

- enhancing and activating various immunological cells in circulation, improving the immunologic function as the main battlefield of killing off the cancer cells in the routing of the metastasis

The stage in which Cancer cell escapes the blood circulation and anchors "target" organ
Third step of anti metastasis

After cancer cell escapes from the blood vessel, it anchors the organ for nidation, forms the new blood vessel and forms the metastatic lesion.

- anti-adherence
- anti-aggregation of blood platelet
- anti cancer embolus
- TG
- Inhibiting angiogenesis factor
- Inhibiting angiogenesis
- Improving immunological regulation
- Improving the immunity of local microenvironment.

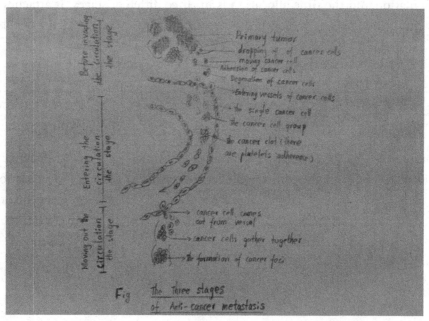

Fig1 The three stages of anti-cancer metastasis

The metastatic lesion is not the terminal. When the metastatic lesion grows up to a certain size, it has the cancer cells separated, intruded and transferred, in this way, it will become a new original place of the cancer cell metastasis. At this moment, the primary lesion and metaststic lesion will become the original place of the ablation and metastasis of the cancer cells via blood metastasis. Therefore, the more and larger the metastatic carcinoma is, the more the cancer cells in the blood circulation are. The number of the immunological cells in the blood circulation of the body of the patient is far insufficient for controlling a large number of cancer cells falling from the carcinoma lesion and entering the blood circulation. The immunologic function of the organism will be severely unbalanced, even the immunologic function will break down, resulting in the hematogenous dissemination. At this time, the organism of the patient will meet with the functional crisis of the immunologic cells. As to how to perfect and deal with this situation, there are only two methods, one is foreign aid and another is endogeny. The foreign aid is the transplantation of stem cell and the endogeny is bioremediation, immunological therapy, genetherapy, molecular biological therapy, treatment by Chinese herbs, Z-C immunologic regulation therapy by Chinese herbs and BRM therapy.

10

Review and Analysis of Clinical Cases of Adjuvant Chemotherapy for Cancer Surgery

- *The cases of cancer postoperative adjuvant chemotherapy failed to prevent recurrence*
- *The cases of cancer postoperative adjuvant chemotherapy failed to prevent metastasis*
- *The cases of chemotherapy to promote immune failure*

In view of the frequent recurrence and metastasis after radical surgery, adjuvant chemotherapy was prevalent after the 1980s. However, postoperative adjuvant chemotherapy prevented recurrence and prevented metastasis, and everyone knew differently. No specific research report has been reported, according to the results of a 5-year follow-up report of patients with adjuvant chemotherapy or radiotherapy for gastric cancer in the UK. The results of adjuvant treatment with mitomycin and fluoropurine bite in the first group of patients in the 1976 British Gastric Cancer Group showed no benefit to postoperative patients. For this purpose, another group of patients underwent r-assisted treatment studies. A prospective randomized controlled group study was performed in 436 patients with gastric adenoma who were staged in the II-ill phase. Postoperative chemotherapy was combined with radiotherapy or mitomycin, doxorubicin, and fluorouridine (MAF). During a 5-year follow-up, a total of 372 patients died, of which 45 died of surgical well-being and 327 died of tumor recurrence. In this randomized study, 145 patients underwent surgery; 153 patients received adjuvant radiotherapy, and the scope of irradiation included the spleen and liver hilar region, with a dose of 4500 cGy; another 138 patients received combination chemotherapy (MAF program), mitomycin 4mg/m^2, doxorubicin 30mg/m^2 and fluorourine 600 mg/m^2, all intravenously, 3 weeks for 1 cycle, A total of 8 cycles are performed.The 2-year overall survival rate of this group of patients was 33% (31% to 35%). The 5-year overall survival rate was 17% (13% - 21%).

Patients who received adjuvant therapy did not have a higher survival rate than those who received surgery alone. For patients who underwent surgery alone, the 5-year survival rate was 20%, surgery plus radiotherapy was 12%, and surgery plus chemotherapy was 19%.

Therefore, surgery is still the standard treatment for stomach pain, and adjuvant treatment should be limited to a certain range of research.

The author has organized, analyzed, evaluated, and reflected on some cases of clinical diagnosis and treatment in the past 10 years (individually asking about medical history, physical examination and treatment, and observation of the whole process).

British Stomach Cancer Group adopted prospective, randomized, controlled grouping research for 436 sdenocarcinoma of stomach patients, whose postoperative staging was phase II to phase III. The 436 postoperative patients were respectively treated by radiation or combined chemotherapy of mitomycin, adriamycin and fluorouracil treatment (MAF). During five-year follow-up, 372 patients died, in which 45 patients died from surgical complications and 327 patients died from tumor relapse. In this randomized grouping research, 145 patients adopted surgical operation. 153 patients accepted adjuvant radiation, and the range of irradiation included hilus lienis and porta hepatis region, also the radiation dose was 4500cGy. Another 138 patients accepted combined chemotherapy (MAF Treatment). Mitomycin was 4mg/m^2; adriamycin was 30 mg/m^2; fluorouracil was 600 mg/m^2. The three drugs were all intravenous injections, and the treatment cycle was 8 cycles, which three weeks were one cycle. Overall two-year survival rate of this group was 33% (31%~35%), and five-year survival rate was 17% (13%~21%). Compared with the survival rate of patients only adopting surgical operation, the survival rate of patients accepting adjuvant treatment had no increase. The five-year survival rate of patients only adopting surgical operation was 20%, rate of surgery and radiation was 12%, and rate of surgery and chemotherapy was 19%.

Thus, surgical operation remains to be the standard treatment for sdenocarcinoma of stomach. The adjuvant treatment measure should be limited within certain field of research.

The writer of this book sorts, analyzes, evaluates and rethinks the following part of the cases (cases with personal inquiry of medical history, medical examination, diagnosis and treat, complete observation) with nearly ten-year personal clinical diagnosis and treatment.

I. Failure Cases of Postoperative Adjuvant Chemotherapy to Arrest Relapse

Case 1 Patient Wei ××, female, fifty, Changsha Hunan, engineer, patient history number: 3300653

Diagnosis: Cystosarcoma phylloides of left breast had serious malignant change and relapse. In July 1996, the patient was found the enlargement of lump in her left breast. The puncture of the lump diagnosed that the lump was fibroma. In October 1996, the left breast was removed. Pathological examination: cystosarcoma phylloides of left breast, level II. Since December 19, 1996, the patient began to accept VAD treatment for chemotherapy and get chemotherapy once every three weeks. The second chemotherapy was on January 16, 1997. Constantly, the third chemotherapy was on February 24, 1997; and then the fourth chemotherapy on March 6, 1997; the fifth chemotherapy on April 8, 1997; the sixth chemotherapy on April 29, 1997. On July 2, 1997, type-B ultrasonic examined that there was a 15mm×12mm sized lump in the similar 9 o'clock position of the right breast. Considering the relapse and metastasis, the patient came to the anti-cancer coordination group (Hubei Group) for outpatient treatment, adopting traditional Chinese and western medicine combination treatment.

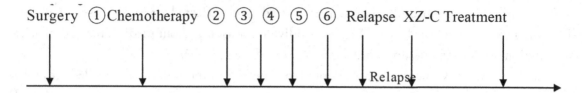

Surgery ①Chemotherapy ② ③ ④ ⑤ ⑥ Relapse XZ-C Treatment

Relapse

Analysis: This patient had one-year postoperative chemotherapies continuously, defining once every month and five days one time. The treatment was standard systematic chemotherapy. But after stopping chemotherapy for two months, the tumor appeared local relapse. That explained that the chemotherapy failed to arrest relapse. It was speculated that chemotherapy might cause the continuing decline of patient's immunity functions beyond retrieval. The tumor lost the immunoregulation and made rest tumor cells set into the cell cycle. Then the tumor was induced. It prompted that long-time continuous chemotherapy must attach importance to protect the host and confront side effects of chemotherapy drugs to avoid the damage for the host. Although chemotherapy killed off tumor cells, it damaged the body at the same time.

Case 2 Patient Yang ×× , female, fifty-four, cadre, Honghu, patient history number: 7201432

Stomach cancer relapsed after surgery. The pain of superior venter had continued for one year. The result of stomachoscopy was stomach cancer. On August 26, 1997, the patient accepted radical operation for stomach cancer. The radical operation was $_2$B1 type. There was a 8mm×5mm sized lump in the lateral side of the lesser curvature of stomach, which caused the pyloric obstruction and enlargement of lymph nodes on the side of the arteria coeliaca. The patient began to accept postoperative chemotherapy after a month. MMC and 5-Fu were seven days one time and the intervals between two times were three weeks. There were total six times in September, October, November, December 1997 and January, February 1998. After that no other treatments were adopted. In January 1999, the patient appeared swallow obstruction and emesis. On February 24, 1999, the patient accepted the stomachoscopy. Front and back of gastric remnant which closed to anastomotic stoma swelled and developed pathological changes. There were mucosal erosion and ulcer. Stomach cancer patient had the postoperative relapse. On March 4, 1999, the patient came to the anti-cancer coordination group (Hubei Group) for XZ-C$_{1+4+2}$ treatment.

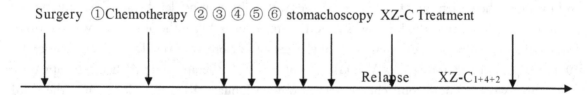

Surgery ①Chemotherapy ② ③ ④ ⑤ ⑥ stomachoscopy XZ-C Treatment

Relapse   XZ-C$_{1+4+2}$

Analysis: This patient had six-time postoperative chemotherapies, defining once every month and seven days one time. The sixth chemotherapy was in February 1998. Until January 1999, the patient appeared swallow obstruction. The result of stomachoscopy was the postoperative relapse of stomach cancer. In this case, the patient had six-time postoperative chemotherapies continuously. It prompted that postoperative adjuvant chemotherapy failed to arrest relapse.

Case 3 Patient Li ××, male, forty-two, Shanxi, cadre, patient history number: 7201427

On November 18, 1997, the patient was found left-liver space occupying lesion through CT in 161 Hospital. On December 2, 1997, the patient accepted the left-liver lateral lobectomy. After 20 days, the patient began to accept postoperative chemotherapy. The chemotherapy drugs were 10mg/dl with intravenous injection and 20mg of hydroxycamptothecine with intravenous injection every other day in two weeks. A course was 15 days. And then the patient needed to repeat the last course after resting 15 days. Before chemotherapy, SGPT was 77μ. After chemotherapy, SGPT was 500μ. In the operation, chemotherapeutic drugs above the chemotherapy pump of portal vein (no chemotherapy pump in the artery) were injected into the organism through the pump. Before the operation, AFP was 200μ. After the operation, AFP was 200μ. In April 1998, the patient accepted the third chemotherapy in the hospital. Chemotherapeutic drugs were injected through the pump. The chemotherapy adopted the high dose pulse therapy, using 6mg of MMC, 200mg of carboplatin and 750mg of 5-Fu. Before chemotherapy, AFP was 180μ. After chemotherapy, AFP was 302μ. On May 19, 1998, the patient accepted the fourth chemotherapy, using the chemotherapy pump as the third time. On June 30, 1998, the patient accepted the fifth chemotherapy with pump. When the AFP was 219μ, it should be detected every other day. On July 28, 1998, the patient accepted the sixth chemotherapy, adopting the high dose pulse therapy through the pump. The reexamination showed that AFP>363. In early August 1998, the examination found that there was a 4cm sized lump under the incision of abdominal wall. On August 27, 1998, the lump was removed in tumor hospital. On September 29, 1998, the patient accepted the seventh chemotherapy with pump. After chemotherapy, the reexamination of type-B ultrasonic, CT and intrahepatic widespread metastasis showed that there were many ball shadows and metastases. In December 1998, the patient accepted hepatic artery embolism and pulmonary intervention in the general hospital of a military region. The examinations found that there were lumps equivalent to the size of an adult fist and infant's head in epigastrium and right abdomen. The lumps were stiff. On March 1, 1999, the patient came to the anti-cancer coordination group (Hubei Group) for outpatient treatment, adopting traditional Chinese and western medicine combination treatment and XZ-C$_{1+4+5}$ series treatment.

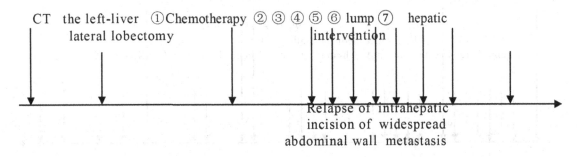

Analysis: This patient suffered from cancer of the liver. After the left-liver lateral lobectomy, the patient had seven-time postoperative chemotherapies continuously, defining once every month. The seventh chemotherapy showed the intrahepatic widespread metastasis and pulmonary metastasis. It prompted that postoperative adjuvant chemotherapy failed to arrest relapse and prevent metastasis.

Case 4 Patient Xiang ××, male, forty-three, cadre, Chongyang, patient history number: 6801345

In June 1994, the disease of this patient was treated as gastroenteritis. Until December, the X-ray examination in city hospital showed that the patient suffered from intestinal obstruction. In early January 1995, the emergency operation explored the disease as a transverse colon tumor. Then the tumor was removed, adopting the end to end anastomosis. Pathological examination showed that the tumor was a malignant tumor. In February, March, April, May, June, July 1995, the patient had six-time postoperative chemotherapies continuously, defining five days one time. In January 1996, the colonic neoplasm of anastomotic stoma was found. The patient accepted the radical excision. At the end of December 1997, the tumor of anastomotic stoma was found again. On March 31, 1998, the patient accepted the palliative excision. In September 1998, another 5.6cm×4.6cm sized lump equivalent to the size of an adult fist was found between stomach and caput pancreatic. On November 24, 1998, the patient underwent an operation again to remove the lump. Those lesser tubercles, such as the omentum, were difficult to be removed completely. And the operation could only remove big ones. In 1996, the patient once accepted four-time postoperative chemotherapies in Tumor Department, defining five days one time. And the patient also took Doxifluridine orally for two months. In April, May 1998, the patient accepted twice chemotherapies. And as well, the patient took two courses of traditional Chinese medicine dispensed by Wang Zhenguo of Shenyang. But the course didn't work. Then the patient took one course of Shijiazhuang Chinese medicine. The course also didn't work. On November 13, 1998, the patient came to the anti-cancer coordination group for outpatient treatment, adopting traditional Chinese and western medicine combination treatment, XZ-C$_{1+4}$ treatment and XZ-C$_2$ treatment. In November 1999, the patient accepted the reexamination, which showed the stable condition.

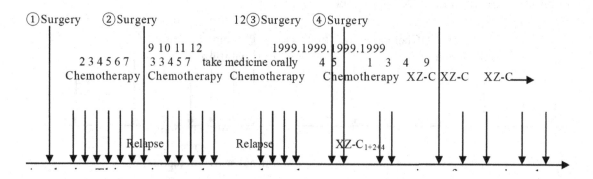

Analysis: This patient underwent the colon cancer operation of removing the tumor. After that, the patient had six-time postoperative chemotherapies continuously, defining once every month and five days one time. Five months later, the colonic neoplasm of anastomotic stoma relapsed and was removed by surgery. During the one year after operation, the patient proceeded with postoperative chemotherapies monthly and continuously. The tumor of anastomotic stoma relapsed and was removed again. The patient proceeded with postoperative chemotherapies. This case prompted that chemotherapy failed to arrest relapse and prevent metastasis. In November 1998, the patient came to the outpatient department for traditional Chinese and western medicine combination treatment, and also took traditional Chinese medicine of XZ-C$_{1+4+2}$ immunoregulation series chronically and continuously. After taking medicine orally, the patient's condition was improved. In November 1999, the patient accepted the reexamination, which showed the stable condition.

Case 5 Patient Li ××, male, fifty, cadre, Hanchuan, patient history number: 5701131

Diagnosis: Rectum cancer relapsed after surgery.

In December 1994, the patient underwent a radical operation for rectum cancer. The operation was Dixon type. The length of rectum cancer lesion was 12cm. The patient had six-time postoperative chemotherapies continuously, defining once every month and seven days one time. The condition was good after operation. On April 30, 1998, the patient accepted the colonoscopy examination. There was a lump at the area of rectum, having 10cm distances to the anus. The 3cm×3cm sized lump had a rugged surface and swelled towards the intracavity. The biopsy of four living tissues showed that the cell had became allotypic gland cell. On June 25, 1998, the patient suffered from the incomplete intestinal obstruction. Then on July 9, 1998, the patient underwent the Hartmann operation and partial cystectomy. The surgery proved it the recurrent rectum cancer, which had involved the bladder. The patient had five-time postoperative radiotherapies for pelvic cavity with accumulated dose of 5000CGY (from October 12, 1998 to November 13, 1998). The patient also had postoperative chemotherapies for one month. The chemotherapy drugs were 5-Fu and calcium leucovorin (five days, once a day). Since the proctoscopy examined the relapse of rectum cancer in May 1998, the patient came to the anti-cancer coordination group for the traditional Chinese medicine treatment of XZ-C immunoregulation series, which was adopted to control the relapse and metastasis. On November 28, 1999, the patient accepted the reexamination. After taking the medicine orally, the patient regained a high spirit, a good appetite and enough physical strength, which showed the stable condition. The patient continued to live normally without any discomfort.

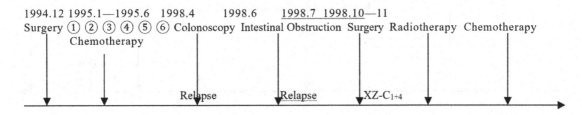

Analysis: After a radical operation for rectum cancer, the patient had six-time postoperative chemotherapies continuously, defining once every month and seven days one time. Two years later, rectum cancer appeared the local recurrence and widespread metastasis. Then the patient continued to accept the chemotherapy, but the rectum cancer relapsed again. It prompted that postoperative adjuvant chemotherapy failed to arrest relapse and prevent metastasis. After the relapse in April 1998, the patient came to the anti-cancer coordination outpatient department for the traditional Chinese medicine treatment of XZ-C$_{1+4}$ immunoregulation series. After taking the medicine orally, the patient's condition was stable and improving. The patient had been persisting in taking the XZ-C medicine for over one year and was being in good health.

Case 6 Patient Luo ××, female, housewife, Gongan county, patient history number: 521020

In September 1994, the patient found a lump in the left breast. The local hospital scanned the lump as a fibroma. In September 1995, because of the enlargement of the lump (5cm×5cm×3cm), the patient underwent a radical operation for breast cancer in the district hospital. Pathology: infiltrating ductal cancer of right breast, ER (+), P.R (+), removal of one subclavicular lymph node and two axillary fusional lymph nodes. After the operation, the patient accepted chemotherapies with CMF treatment for one week. On December 6, 1995, the patient accepted chemotherapies with CAF treatment for one week. On December 26, 1995, the patient accepted chemotherapies with CAF treatment for one week again. From February 5, 1996 to March 30, the patient accepted radiotherapies. In August 1996, the patient continued to accept two courses of chemotherapies, defining three weeks of one course. In September 1997, a lump was found in the right axilla. There were tubercles under the prethoracic skin again. The breast cancer appeared relapse and metastasis. Then the patient came to the anti-cancer coordination outpatient department for the traditional Chinese medicine treatment of XZ-C immunoregulation series. On January 4, 1998, the patient began to take XZ-C medicine during the outpatient treatment. After taking 45-day medicine, the patient's condition kept stable. In October 1998, the patient accepted the reexamination in the outpatient department, which showed the stable condition. There was a tubercle equivalent to the size of the little finger in the top part of right axilla. Above this tubercle, there was another tubercle equivalent to the size of a rice grain. But it had no more growth.

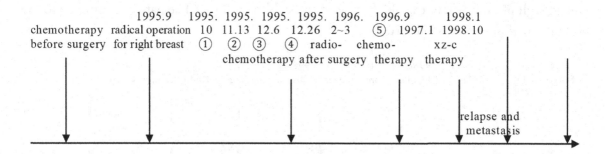

Analysis: The patient suffered from the breast cancer. Before the surgery, the patient accepted one-week chemotherapies. After the surgery, the patient accepted postoperative chemotherapies, defining once every month and one-week one time. But the treatment failed to prevent metastasis, diffusion and progression. In January 1998, the patient came to the outpatient department and took 10-month traditional Chinese medicine of immunoregulation. The patient's condition was stable. The breast cancer had no more progress. The general condition was improving.

Case 7 Patient Yang ××, female, fifty, Hankou, technical cadre, patient history number: 54001079

Diagnosis: Rectal adenocarcinoma relapsed after surgery.

In June 1996, the patient was diagnosed with rectum cancer for diarrhea. On July 11, 1996, the patient underwent a radical low anterior resection operation for rectum cancer. In the operation, the tumor located under the reflection, which was 5cm×4cm and invaded the muscular layer. The lymph node under the mesentery developed obvious enlargement. The patient recovered well from the operation. Nine days after the operation, the patient accepted chemotherapies of 5-Fu and MMC series. After leaving hospital, the patient took Mifulong orally. On October 4, 1996, the patient accepted chemotherapies in a tumor hospital and then left it. From August 17, 1996 to October 5, the patient accepted three courses of chemotherapies with ELF treatment. From January 14, 1997 to February 3, the patient accepted the third chemotherapies in a tumor hospital of MMC and 5-Fu series. After the chemotherapy, the patient began the attack of diarrhea more than ten times every day. From May 1997 to July 1997, the patient took Mifulong orally. On February 4, 1998, the patient had a return visit for the rectal examination. In the area of the anastomotic stoma, the tubercle could be touched. The rectum cancer relapsed. The patient accepted eight chemotherapies again and 21 radiotherapies. Then the patient had hematuria and diarrhea. It showed that the patient suffered from the radioactive cystitis and radioactive rectitis.

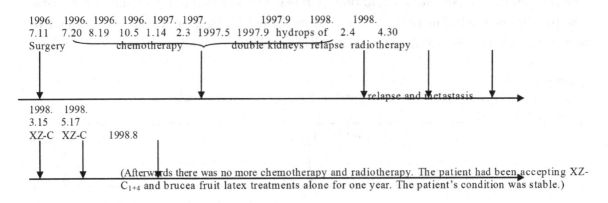

(Afterwards there was no more chemotherapy and radiotherapy. The patient had been accepting XZ-C$_{1+4}$ and brucea fruit latex treatments alone for one year. The patient's condition was stable.)

Analysis: This case was the rectal adenocarcinoma. After the radical operation, the patient accepted chemotherapies continuously. On February 4, 1998, the rectum cancer relapsed in the area of the anastomotic stoma. The patient had accepted continuous and multiple chemotherapies, involving intravenous chemotherapies and oral chemotherapy drugs. But it failed to arrest the relapse of rectum cancer in the area of the anastomotic stoma. After finding the relapse, the patient accepted radiotherapies and chemotherapies continuously again. These treatments also evoked the radioactive cystitis and other complicating diseases. The treatments failed to prevent the progression of recurrent cancer.

On March 15, 1998, the patient came to the anti-cancer coordination group for outpatient treatment, simply adopting the traditional Chinese medicine of XZ-C immunoregulation series and brucea fruit latex for enema. After taking the medicine, the patient's general condition was getting better. And the spirit and appetite were improving. The patient had chronically been taking the traditional Chinese medicine of XZ-C immunoregulation series for eighteen months. The condition of illness was stable. The tumor had been controlled, and it was stable with no more progression. The patient's condition was getting better markedly.

Case 8 Patient Xu ××, female, fifty-six, Macheng, patient history number: 7401472

Diagnosis: Lymph nodes of the left ventral groove metastasized. The adenocarcinoma of anal canal relapsed.

For the blood-stained stool, three blood examinations showed that the patient suffered from the cancer of anus. On February 25, 1997, the patient underwent a Miles-type radical operation for cancer of anal canal. The appendages of ambo-uterus were removed. Lymph nodes of the left perineum and ventral groove were cleaned. The patient had six-time postoperative chemotherapies. The first chemotherapy was on May 24, 1997 with MMC+5-Fu treatment. The second chemotherapy was on July 2, 1997. The third chemotherapy was on August 13, 1997. The fourth chemotherapy was on September 17, 1997. The fifth chemotherapy was on February 8, 1998. The sixth chemotherapy was on November 15, 1998. Since September 1997, the patient began to have the feeling of swell, distention, burn and urodynia in the area of anus. On April 14, 1999, the detected value of CEA was 5.8mg/ml. On April 16, 1999, the patient came to the anti-cancer coordination group for the traditional Chinese medicine treatment of immunoregulation. The patient had the feeling of swell, ache and tenderness in the area of anus. There was a very high chance that exfoliated survival cancer cells had relapsed.

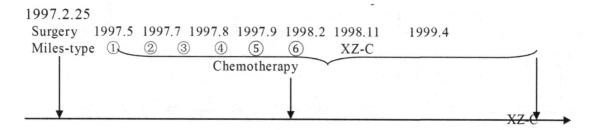

Analysis: After the Miles-type radical operation for cancer of anal canal, the patient accepted chemotherapies of six courses continuously. In September 1997, the patient began to have the feeling of ache and tenderness in the area of anus. And the feeling of pain became doubly intense. It was obvious that exfoliated survival cancer cells were proliferating and relapsing. The poisonous drugs for cancers cells in continuous chemotherapies failed to totally destroy these exfoliated survival cancer cells. Thus, these cancer cells revived again, proliferating and relapsing in partial place.

Case 9 Patient Xiong ××, male, forty-two, worker, Wuhan, patient history number: 6501291

Diagnosis: Rectum cancer relapsed after surgery.

In March 1998, for the blood-stained stool, the disease of this patient was treated as "hemorrhoid". In May 1998, the proctoscop biopsy examination showed that the patient suffered from rectum cancer. On May 29, 1998, the patient underwent a Miles-type radical operation for rectum cancer. The postoperative plug was poorly differentiated rectum cancer. The cancer cells had invaded to the full-thickness of intestinal wall, involving the adipose tissue around the rectum. The lymph nodes around the rectum also had metastases (16/17). The patient accepted the postoperative chemotherapies. The first chemotherapy was in June 1998, adopting the MMC+5-Fu treatment for five days. In July 1998, the patient accepted chemotherapies for twelve days (pelvic cavity, front and back of abdomen) with twenty-four times. And then the second chemotherapy was in September 1998, adopting the MMC+5-Fu treatment for six days. The third chemotherapy was in November 1999, adopting the same drugs as the second chemotherapy for five days. On November 2, 1998, the patient accepted the reexamination of type-B ultrasonic. There was no abnormality in the pelvic cavity. In February 1999, the patient began to feel pain in the area of anus. The examination of type-B ultrasonic still showed no abnormality. In March, the CT examination showed that there was a lump in the deep part of pelvic cavity (the area of anus). On March 15, 1999, the patient accepted the radiotherapies of pelvic cavity for fifteen days. In the following five days, the patient had the chemotherapies. And then the patient proceeded with radiotherapies for six times. During the radiotherapies and chemotherapies, the patient was treated by XZ-C4 to fight against the toxic side effect and protect the chest and marrow for hematopoiesis and immunization. There was no untoward effect in the whole process. Since November 1998, the patient had been using the XZ-C series for the traditional Chinese medicine treatment of immunoregulation. The condition of the illness was stable and getting better.

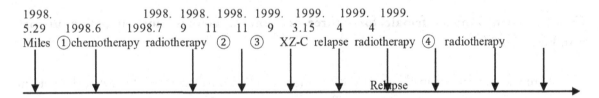

Analysis: After the Miles-type radical operation for rectum cancer, the patient accepted chemotherapies and radiotherapies continuously. Three months later, the CT examination showed that there was a lump in the deep part of pelvic cavity. The patient began to have the feeling of ache in the area of anus. The rectum cancer relapsed in partial place. It prompted that postoperative continuous chemotherapy failed to prevent the local recurrence.

Case 10 Patient Zhang ×× , female, forty-four, married, Hankou, patient history number: 7101407

Diagnosis: Infiltrating ductal cancer of right breast relapsed after surgery.

Authors: Xu Ze (China) ; Xu Jie(China) ; Bin Wu(America)

In October 1997, the patient underwent the radical operation of mastocarcinoma for breast cancer (above 5m²). Twenty days later, the patient accepted intravenous chemotherapies for eight days with CMF treatment. In December after leaving hospital, the patient accepted radiotherapies for twenty-five times. After that, the patient accepted the chemotherapies again. In February, March, April, May and June 1998, the patient accepted chemotherapies for six times, defining once every month. In April 1998, at the lower end of the incision, a tubercle about the size of a bean could be touched. Since then, the skin tubercles grew more and more. Now eczematoid lesion was diffusing around the skin incision, and the cancer cells had been metastasizing through the whole body. There was a cauliflower-shaped ulcer (3cm×3cm) in the middle part of incisional scar. On February 3, 1999, the patient came to the anti-cancer coordination group for outpatient treatment, adopting the traditional Chinese medicine treatment of XZ-C immunoregulation series and brucea fruit latex treatment. The condition of the illness was stable.

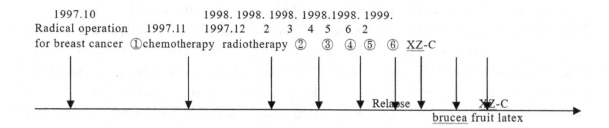

Analysis: After the operation for breast cancer, the patient accepted chemotherapies and radiotherapies continuously. Six months after the operation, when the patient was accepting chemotherapies, the cancer relapsed in partial places and the cancer cells metastasized through the whole body. It prompted that postoperative continuous radiotherapies and chemotherapies failed to prevent relapse and metastasis.

Case 11 Patient Yang ××, female, forty-three, accountant, Henan Luoshan, patient history number: 521024

There was red mucus in the stool for one month. Then on December 23, 1997, the patient accepted the fibercoloscope examination. There was an irregularly shaped new growth (3cm×5cm) at the ascending colon of the blinding end, which had 100cm to the fibercoloscope. The surface of the new growth was rugged and anabrotic. The pathological test proved it villoglandular adenocarcinoma. On December 30, 1997, the patient underwent the radical operation for colon cancer to remove the right hemicolon. In the operation, it could be found that there was a 4cm×4cm sized lump in the juncture between the blind gut and the ascending colon. The lymph nodes of the mesocolic root enlarged. The cancer cells had no metastases to the liver. Pathological test showed that villoglandular adenocarcinoma (part of mucinous adenocarcinoma) had invaded to the full-thickness of intestinal wall. Twenty-two lymph nodes had no metastases. The patient accepted postoperative chemotherapies for six times, defining once every month. The first chemotherapy was on November 26, 1998, continuing for eight days with FAP and hydroxycamptothecine. The second time started from February 12, 1998. A month later, the third time proceeded. The fourth time was on April 25, 1998 with FP treatment. The fifth time was on May 27, 1998. And the sixth time was on June 27, 1998. The chemotherapy continued for eight days. The patient had mild side effects. The white blood cell count (WBC) was 2100. On January 4, 1999, the patient accepted chemotherapies for ten days with MMC and hydroxycamptothecine. From February 1, 1999 to February 10, the patient accepted the tenth chemotherapy. In April 1999, the fibercoloscope reexamination showed the anastomosis ulcer of the colon. And the cancer relapsed in the anastomotic stoma. Then the patient came to the anti-cancer coordination group for outpatient treatment, adopting traditional Chinese and western medicine combination treatment, i.e. XZ-C$_{1+4}$ and brucea fruit latex. The condition of the illness was stable and getting better.

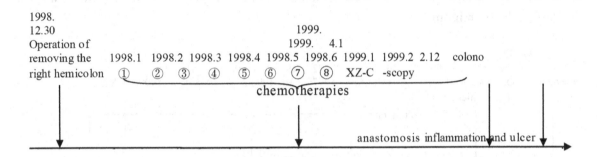

Analysis: After the radical excision for adenocarcinoma of ascending colon, the patient accepted chemotherapies for eight courses, defining one course of one month and eight days of one course. After the eighth course, the fibercoloscope reexamination showed the recurrence of anastomotic stoma. It prompted that postoperative continuous chemotherapies with eight lengthy courses still failed to prevent relapse.

Case 12 Patient Fu ××, male, twenty-four, demobilized soldier, Henan, Hu Aibin. patient history number: 8201626

Diagnosis: The carcinoma of colon relapsed after surgery.

Medical History: In February 1996, the abdominal pain was falsely diagnosed as appendicitis. Then the patient underwent the operation of removing the appendix. Pathological examination of appendicitis showed no inflammation. After the operation, the patient still felt pain in the abdominal region with recurrent paroxysmal pain. And it was treated as the spasmolysis of intestinal adhesion. Until December 1996, the patient underwent the operation of abdominal laparotomy in 153 Hospital of Zhengzhou because of intestinal obstruction. The operation showed that there was a tumor in the right hemicolon. Then the patient underwent the radical excision for right hemicolon. The pathological report was as follows. The patient suffered from the carcinoma of colon. Half month after the operation, the patient began to accept chemotherapies. The first chemotherapy started from January 1997 and continued for five days with the intravenous injection (iv). And the chemotherapy drugs were 5-Fu+cis-platinum+MMC. The second chemotherapy was in March 1997. The third time was in May. The forth time was in August. The fifth time was in October. The sixth time was in December 1997. In the following year, the patient accepted the chemotherapy every three months. The seventh time was in March 1998. The eighth time was in June 1998. The ninth time was in September 1998. The tenth time was in December 1998. (In 1997, there was one time every two months with a total of six times. In 1998, there was one time every three months with a total of four times.) The eleventh time was in October 1999. In January 1999, the patient began to feel pain and constantly pain in the lumbosacral portion. In August 1999, the patient began to feel pain in the abdominal region and have the abdominal tympania. And there was mucus in the stool. On November 14, 1999, the patient came to the anti-cancer coordination outpatient department for XZ-C$_{1+3+4}$ treatment. On November 15, 1999, the patient underwent a colonoscopy in the general hospital of Chinese People's Liberation Army (301 hospital). The examination showed that there was a recurrent tumor in the region, having 10cm to 30cm distances to the anus. Pathological examination showed that this tumor was the anaplastic adenocarcinoma.

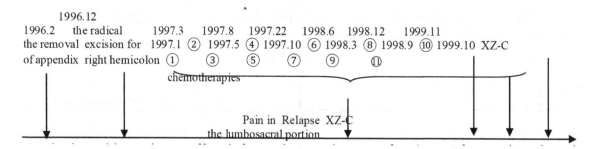

Analysis: This patient suffered from the carcinoma of colon. After undergoing the radical excision for right hemicolon, the patient accepted chemotherapies for eleven times continuously, defining two courses of one month in the first year after the operation and one course of three months in the second year after the operation. Until the tenth chemotherapy, the patient began to feel pain in the abdominal region. Retroperitoneal metastases appeared. The left colorectal cancer relapsed. Relapse and metastasis appeared while the chemotherapies were continuing. It prompted that postoperative adjuvant chemotherapy failed to arrest relapse and prevent metastasis.

II. Failure Cases of Postoperative Adjuvant Chemotherapy to Prevent Metastasis

Case 13 Patient, Xu ××, male, fifty-two, peasant, Xinzhou, patient history number: 6901374

Diagnosis: The hepatic metastases happened after the operation of carcinoma of anal canal.

The patient suffered from the carcinoma of anal canal. On September 23, 1997, the patient underwent the Miles-type radical operation. The tumor had 2cm from the anus, having the size of 3cm×3cm×2cm. The pathology was squamous cell carcinoma of anal canal. The patient accepted the postoperative chemotherapies once a month. There were five days per month for intravenous injection with carboplatin+5-Fu in October and November 1997. There were also five days per month for intravenous injection with MMC+5-Fu in December 1997, January 1998, February 1998 and March 1998. In April and May 1998, the patient switched to the oral route of Ftorafur-207 tablets. In June 1998, the type-B ultrasonic showed no abnormality. But on January 8, 1999, the type-B ultrasonic showed that there were multiple occupying nidi in the liver. The biggest nidus had the size of 8.2cm×8.6cm, diagnosed as intrahepatic metastases and retroperitoneal lymphatic metastases. There were several lymph nodes with the size of 2.1cm×0.5cm.

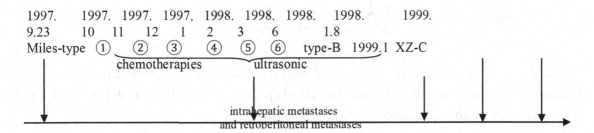

Analysis: This patient underwent the Miles-type operation. And the operation means was right. After the operation, the patient accepted chemotherapies once a month for six times continuously. Then the patient took the chemotherapy drugs orally for two months. The carboplatin, MMC and 5-Fu failed to prevent carcinomatous metastases. The tumor was the carcinoma of anal canal. But the first metastasis was hepatic metastasis. It prompted that continuous and systematical chemotherapies after the operation still failed to prevent hepatic metastases.

Case 14 Patient Yu ××, male, fifty-seven, worker, Nanchang, patient history number: 6901366

On October 22, 1995, the patient underwent the Miles-type radical operation for rectum cancer in a central hospital of Nanchang. After operation, the patient accepted the first chemotherapy was on December 5, 1995 with intravenous injection of 1000mg of 5-Fu once a day (d_1, d_2, d_3, d_4) and intravenous injection of 6mg of MMC (d_1). The second time was on February 2, 1996 with the same FM treatment as the first time. The third time was on March 18, 1996 with the same treatment. The fourth time was on May 24, 1996. The fifth time was on August 14, 1996. The sixth time was on September 14, 1996. All of the chemotherapies adopted the FM treatment. After the chemotherapies, the patient underwent the CT examination. On December 28, 1998, the report showed three points: ①fatty liver and metastatic liver cancer, ②colorectal cancer metastasis, ③polycystic kidney and calculus of kidney. On December 25, 1998, the type-B ultrasonic found the space occupying lesion of liver.

On December 30, 1998, the patient came to the anti-cancer coordination group for outpatient treatment with XZ-C$_{4+5+3}$. The examination showed that a lump in the form of bar could be touched in the right liver and the lump was hard. On January 20, 1999, the type-B ultrasonic in a central hospital of Nanchang found several tumors of unequal size about 4cm×2.1cm, 2.2cm×1.8cm and 2.0cm×1.7cm in the liver. There was a metastatic liver cancer with the size of 3.0cm×2.9cm in the right liver. On February 20, 1999, after taking the XZ-C$_{1+4}$, the patient's condition was stable and the patient regained a high spirit, a good appetite. The liver was functioning normally. The patient could walk on the street as a normal people. The symptom had an obvious improvement.

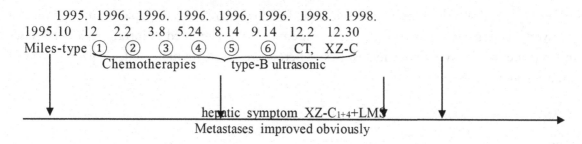

Analysis: After the radical operation of rectum cancer, the patient accepted continuous chemotherapies for six courses. One year later, the hepatic metastases happened. It prompted that systematical chemotherapies failed to prevent metastases.

Case 15 Patient Guo ××, male, thirty-six, teacher, Wuhan, patient history number: 7201425

In October 1996, the patient suffered from gastric bleeding. Then the stomachoscopy showed that the patient suffered from the stomach cancer. The patient underwent the total gastrectomy in a general hospital. Two months after the operation, the chemotherapies started. The patient accepted once every two months, defining ten days of one time. The chemotherapy drugs were MMC and 5Fu with intravenous injection. This course lasted for one year (six times). In the second year, the patient accepted once every half year. The chemotherapies in 1998 were carried out once every three or four months. In September 1998, the patient accepted one time. Every time before the chemotherapy, the patient needed to undergo the examination of type-B ultrasonic. If the type-B ultrasonic showed that there was a problem, the type-B ultrasonic would be switched to CT. The patient underwent the CT examinations for five times successively, and the CT was strengthened. After the last chemotherapy in September 1998, CT showed that the cancer cells were metastasizing to liver and retroperitoneum. Then the patient underwent the photon knife (X-knife) treatment for one time and the interventional chemotherapy for hepatic vessels embolism. In October 1998, the sclera of the patient turned yellow. The CT showed that the nubbly lump of caput pancreatic was oppressing the bile duct. Then the patient underwent the radiotherapies continuously for three times in October, November 1998 and January 1999. The doses at a time were 4000 dela. The patient had an intense reaction with bad physiques and vomiting, and couldn't feed at all. The patient couldn't undergo it and stopped the treatment. On February 28, 1999, the patient came to the outpatient department of anti-cancer coordination group for traditional Chinese and western medicine combination treatment. At that time, the patient had been bedridden. The patient was not able to take in any food for the repeated nausea and vomiting. After taking the XZ-C drugs, the patient was getting better.

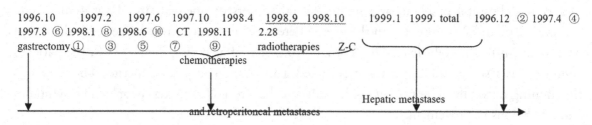

Analysis: After the total gastrectomy, the patient underwent the continuous chemotherapies and radiotherapies for a long time. After the last chemotherapy in September 1998, the CT reexamination showed the hepatic metastases and retroperitoneal metastases. It prompted that continuous and long-term treatments still failed to prevent metastases, even resulting in the failure of immunologic system and threatening the patient's life.

Case 16 Patient Cao ×× , male, thirty-five, married, peasant, Hanchuan, patient history number: 470928

Diagnosis: The hepatic metastases happened after the operation of stomach cancer.

On June 28, 1996, the pre-operative diagnosis in the People's Hospital of Hanchuan certified it as the ulcer of gastric angles. The property of the illness was yet to be investigated. The patient underwent the massive resection of the stomach and the resection of great epiploon. The operation was B1-type anastomosis. The postoperative pathological report showed it the sdenocarcinoma of stomach. The cancer cells had invaded the full-thickness of stomach wall with lymphatic metastases of lesser curvature side (4/4). The lymph nodes of greater curvature side had reactive hyperplasia. The patient underwent the postoperative chemotherapies for four times in July, August, September and October 1996, defining once a month and three days every time. The chemotherapy drugs were 5-F and MMC. In September 1997, after the half month of swelling pain in right upper abdomen, the type-B ultrasonic and CT prompted that there were several low-density shadows in the right and left lobe of liver. Those were metastatic hepatic tumors and could be touched below the right costal margin of 3cm with pressing tender. On September 30, 1997, the patient underwent the interventional chemotherapy for hepatic artery. On October 5, 1997, the patient came to the anti-cancer coordination outpatient department, adopting the Z-C series for the traditional Chinese medicine treatment of immunoregulation. After taking the medicine orally, the patient regained a high spirit, a good appetite and enough physical strength. The lump below the right costal margin became soft and narrowing.

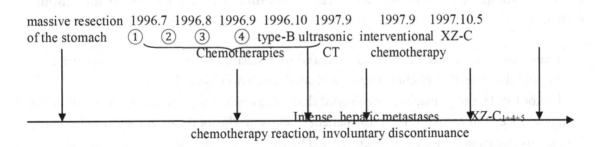

Analysis: After the operation of stomach cancer, the patient underwent the continuous chemotherapies for four times, defining once a month and three days every time. One year after the last chemotherapy, the CT reexamination showed that there were several metastatic lesions in the right and left lobe of liver. It prompted that postoperative adjuvant chemotherapies still failed to prevent metastases.

Case 17 Patient Li ××, male, fifty-five, Huangshi, second-grade actor, patient history number: 2700530

Diagnosis: The cancer cells metastasized to pancreas after the operation of stomach cancer.

In October 1995, the patient suffered from the epigastric discomfort. In November, the stomachoscopy in Huangshi Hospital diagnosed it as the stomach cancer. On November 27, 1995, the patient underwent the massive resection of the stomach. After the operation, the patient accepted five courses of chemotherapies with one course per month. In early May 1996, the last course ended. On June 4, 1996, the CT reexamination showed the space occupying lesion of pancreas. The patient began to have the abdominal distension and bad appetite. Then the patient came to the anti-cancer coordination group for outpatient treatment, adopting the XZ-C$_{1+4+2}$ series for the traditional Chinese medicine treatment of immunoregulation. After taking the medicine orally, the patient regained a high spirit, a good appetite.

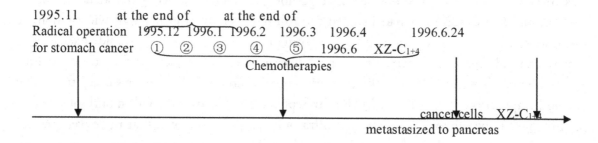

Analysis: After the radical operation of stomach cancer, the patient accepted five courses of chemotherapies with one course per month. After the five courses, the patient underwent the CT reexamination, finding the space occupying lesion of pancreas and metastatic carcinoma of pancreas. It prompted that postoperative chemotherapies still failed to prevent postoperative carcinomatous metastases.

Case 18 Patient Li ××, female, forty-five, Guangshui, teacher, patient history number: 6701324

Diagnosis: The stomach cancer relapsed and metastasized to ovary after the operation. The middle and down section of choledochus had solid space occupying lesions.

In April 1998, the stomachoscopy showed that there was a new growth in the body of stomach with bulb ulcer. On April 20, 1998, the patient underwent the total gastrectomy and lienectomy. Esophagus and empty intestine were connected by the end-to-side anastomosis. The pathological test showed that the patient suffered from the mucinous adenocarcinoma of stomach. The cancer cells had invaded the full-thickness of stomach wall with lymphatic metastases of lesser curvature side. On May 13, 1998, the patient accepted the first chemotherapy, adopting 1000mg of 5-Fu with five-day intravenous injections. On the first day the chemotherapy drugs were added with 10mg of Mitomycin. On June 3, 1998, the patient accepted the second chemotherapy with 10mg of Mitomycin. The third time was on July 1, 1998. The fourth time was on July 29, 1998. The fifth time was on September 9, 1998. The reexamination found the relapse. On December 24, 1998, the type-B ultrasonic showed the cancer of biliary duct and ovarian metastasis. On December 26, 1998, the patient came to the anti-cancer coordination group for outpatient treatment, adopting the XZ-C series for the traditional Chinese medicine treatment of immunoregulation. After taking the medicine orally, the symptom was improving, and the condition of the illness was getting better.

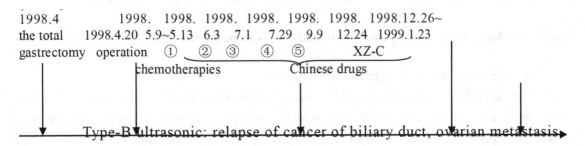

Analysis: This patient suffered from the mucinous adenocarcinoma of stomach and underwent the total gastrectomy. After the operation, the patient accepted the chemotherapies once a month with five days per time. After the fifth chemotherapy, the type-B ultrasonic found the relapse of cancer of biliary duct and ovarian metastasis. It prompted that postoperative adjuvant chemotherapies still failed to arrest relapse and prevent metastasis.

Case 19 Patient Li xx, female, thirty-seven, worker, Yingcheng, patient history number: 7401473

Diagnosis: The rectum cancer cells metastasized to ovary after the operation.

Since 1997, the stool had been being with the blood. In June 1998, the colonoscopy showed it as the rectum cancer. On July 9, 1998, the patient underwent the anterior resection of the rectum (Dixon-type, anastomat). There were six-time postoperative chemotherapies. The first time was on July 27, 1998 with carboplatin and 5-Fu. The second time was on September 6, 1998. The third time was on October 2, 1998. The fourth time was on November 19, 1998. The fifth time was on December 25, 1998. The sixth time was on January 31, 1999.

On April 16, 1999, the patient came to the anti-cancer coordination group for outpatient treatment with the XZ-C series. In May 1999, the CT examination showed the rectum cancer cells metastasized to bilateral ovaries.

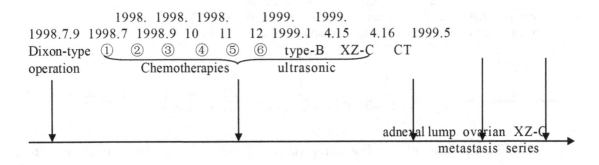

Analysis: After the operation of rectum cancer, the patient accepted continuous chemotherapies for six courses. Three months after the last course, the type-B ultrasonic and CT found that rectum cancer cells metastasized to bilateral ovaries. It prompted that such continuous and long-term chemotherapies still failed to prevent metastases.

III. Cases of Chemotherapy Accelerating the Failure of Immunologic Function

Case 20 Patient, Xu ××, male, forty-two, cadre, Wuhan, patient history number: 420836

Diagnosis: Lung cancer of right middle lobe

In February 1997, fluoroscopy of chest showed no abnormity. Because of the home decorating, the patient had contacted the marble powder bed for about one month. Then this patient began to have a complaint of the chest. On June 1, 1997, X-ray chest film showed the atelectasis of right lung. On June 13, 1997, the CT reported the lung cancer of median lobe and metastases of hilar lymph nodes. The examination of bronchofiberscope showed that each bronchus of the right side became narrower. The brushing biopsy showed it as the adenocarcinoma cell. Right now, the patient had no cough and emptysis. There was a lymph node about the size of fingertip in the right neck region. On June 13, 1997, the patient underwent the interventional therapy for one time. Because of the intense reaction, there was no more interventional therapy. On July 25, 1997, the patient began to accept chemotherapies for two times. The first time adopted the intravenous injection with a large dose of Adriamycin, Cyclophosphane, Cis-platinum and **Xierke**. On August 9, the white blood cell count (WBC) was 1100. Then the patient accepted the blood transfusion, adding with injections of interleukin-2, tumor necrosis factor and interferon. The second time was on August 20. The chemotherapy drugs were same as the first time with intravenous injection. On September 10, X-ray chest film showed no obvious pathological change. On September 11, the patient left the hospital. On October 10, 1997, Emission Computed Tomography (ECT) showed widespread metastatic tumor of bone of the whole body. On October 13, 1997, X-ray chest film showed the lung cancer of double lungs. The lesions increased significantly as compared with the past. After undergoing the reinforced chemotherapies of two courses, the lesions of double lungs spread. The cancer cells quickly metastasized to skeletons of the whole body. The immunologic function broke down. By the end of October 1997, the patient died from the failure of immunologic function.

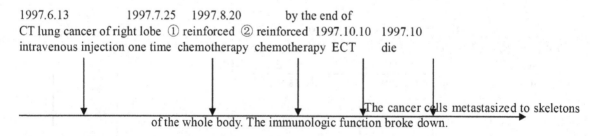

1997.6.13   1997.7.25   1997.8.20   by the end of
CT lung cancer of right lobe ① reinforced ② reinforced 1997.10.10 1997.10
intravenous injection one time chemotherapy chemotherapy ECT   die

The cancer cells metastasized to skeletons of the whole body. The immunologic function broke down.

Analysis: This patient suffered from lung cancer of right middle lobe. The left lung had carcinomatous metastasis. So the patient couldn't accept the operation. Since July 1997, the patient accepted the reinforced chemotherapies of two courses with four kinds of drugs. The patient began to vomit and couldn't feed at all. After the treatment, the immunologic function of the patient broke down. Emission Computed Tomography (ECT) showed that there were several dozen osseous metastases in the whole body. It prompted: ① the reinforced chemotherapies failed to prevent metastases. ② the reinforced chemotherapies severely suppressed the immunity, which led to the severe failure of immunologic function. The host lost the immune surveillance. The cancer cells immediately spread to the whole body. The osseous metastases resulted in the failure of immunologic function and shortened this patient's life.

Case 21 Patient Feng ××, female, fifty-one, Xiangfan, doctor, patient history number: 4900972

Diagnosis: After the operation of the breast cancer, the cancer cells metastasized to bones, liver and brain.

In February 1995, the patient underwent the modified radical mastectomy for the lump in the right breast. The patient suffered from the metastatic carcinoma of axillary lymph nodes (3/6). Pathology: infiltrating ductal cancer became partly hard. On February 19, 1995, the patient accepted the chemotherapy with the drugs of Adriamycin and Cyclophosphamide. On April 28, 1995, the patient transferred to Wuhan for eleven cycles of chemotherapies with CMF treatment. On May 21, 1996, the CMF treatment was switched to Xierke treatment in the eleventh cycle. The arrest of bone marrow became obvious. The white blood cell count (WBC) dropped to 300! Transfusion of 20g of leucocytes eventually made it come back to the normal value. The doctor gave express order that the patient couldn't accept the treatment after leaving hospital. On June 4, 1996, the Ct reexamination found metastatic carcinoma of the ninth rib. Then the patient accepted the radiotherapies without any chemotherapy. On July 7, 1997, the type-B ultrasonic found the metastatic carcinoma of liver. There was a tumor about the size of 3.2cm×3.9cm in the right anterior lobe of liver. The MRI and CT examinations diagnosed it falsely as radioactive hepatic lesion. On July 17, 1997, the angiography proved it as the metastatic carcinoma of liver. On July 28, 1997, the patient underwent the resection of the right anterior lobe of liver. And the patient was inserted a catheter into the hepatic artery for implantation of the drug pump. The chemotherapy drugs of epirubicin, cis-platinum and 5-Fu had been pumped successively for four times. On November 10, 1997, the type-B ultrasonic found that there were a metastatic carcinoma about the size of 3.4cm×3.3cm in the right lobe of liver and another metastatic carcinoma about the size of 1.7cm×1.9cm in the right anterior lobe of liver. The patient couldn't undergo the surgery, radiotherapy or chemotherapy any more. That was because none of the three treatments could prevent metastasis and extension. On November 16, 1997, the patient came to the anti-cancer coordination group for outpatient treatment, adopting the XZ-C series for the traditional Chinese medicine complex treatment of immunoregulation. After taking the medicine, the patient regained a high spirit, a good appetite. The general condition was improving. On March 17, 1998, MRI showed that there were multiple occupying nidi inside the calvarium. The cancer cells were metastasizing to the brain. Then the patient accepted the reinforced chemotherapies. After a course of reinforced chemotherapies, the patient gradually faded away.

Authors: Xu Ze (China) ; Xu Jie(China) ; Bin Wu(America)

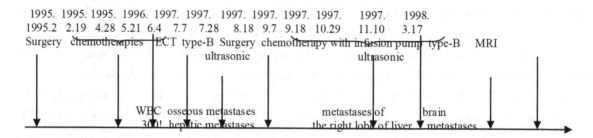

Analysis:

(1) After the operation of breast cancer, the patient accepted the continuous chemotherapies, starting with short-course chemotherapies and proceeding with the eleven courses of chemotherapies. And then, the patient was injected with the chemotherapy drugs by the infusion pump. Although the patient continuously accepted the chemotherapies and other treatments without a stop, the cancer still ignored those treatments, slowly and gradually making the distant metastases through the whole body. Why did so many treatments fail to stop metastases and extensions? What kind of role and status did those chemotherapy anti-cancer drugs play and have in this case? The chemotherapies didn't produce the due effect, because after the chemotherapy the cancer cells immediately metastasized to bones, liver.

(2) The chemotherapy suppressed the immunologic function and marrow hematopoietic function. The question was whether the suppression would promote osseous metastases. The reinforced chemotherapies of this case once made WBC reduce to 300. The body's immunological function suffered the severe suppression. The cancer cells lost the immune surveillance and would inevitably have the further multiplications, extensions and metastases.

(3) Why were the chemotherapies of this case useless? The question was whether the chemotherapy drugs had the drug tolerance. If having the tolerance, the chemotherapy drugs of more than one year were totally useless. The drugs didn't produce the due effect on cancer cells. On the contrary, the normal cells of visceral organs in the patient's body, especially the cells of immune organ (Marrow was the central immune organ), ceaselessly suffered form the damage. Then the ability of the body resistance and immunological function severely fell off. It promoted multiplications, extensions and metastases of cancer cells. The chemotherapy not only failed to achieve the therapeutic effect, but also conversely had the adverse effect on attacking the ability of the body resistance and promoting the metastases and multiplications of the cancer cells.

(4) Why were the continuous chemotherapies of this case useless? The question was whether the selected joint chemotherapy drugs were not sensitive to the cancer cells of this patient. (The anti-cancer drugs couldn't accept drug sensitive test as the antibiotic. Thus the drugs were selected according to the experience with certain blindness.) When doctors couldn't get the curative effect, they would increase the dose, intensify the chemotherapy or switch to use the better chemotherapy drugs. In this way, it would produce the more

202

severe immunological suppression, result the failure of immunological function and lead to the further multiplications of the cancer cells, which the cancer cells would present the multiplication like the geometrical logarithm. But the chemotherapy drugs couldn't increase exponentially with the toxic side effect. Thus the increasing speed and quantity of chemotherapy drugs would never be able to catch up those of cancer cells. So the continuous chemotherapies still failed to control metastases and extensions.

Case 22 Patient Lu ××, female, forty-three, shop employee, Changsha, patient history number: 4300857

Diagnosis: The patient suffered from the carcinoma simplex of left breast. The cancer cells had metastasized to the back bone, pelvis and liver.

Medical History: (Omission).

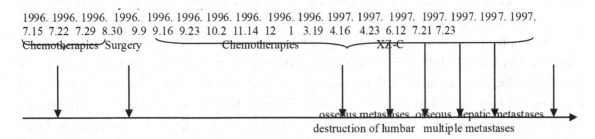

Analysis: This patient accepted the preoperative and postoperative chemotherapies continuously and chronically. After the operation, the patient accepted the chemotherapy once a month, defining five days every time. During the five months after the operation, there were over forty times of radiotherapies and eight times of chemotherapies. The patient underwent continuous multiple CT scans and ceaselessly continuous chemotherapies. But after eight months the cancerous protuberance widely metastasized and spread to skeletons of the whole body. Every time the patient accepted the radiotherapy or chemotherapy, she had to suffer the suppression, bone marrow suppression and the attack to the organisms of the body. The long-term and continuous chemotherapies were essentially the chronic and continuous attack to the immunologic function. The immunologic function of organisms and marrow hematopoietic function suffered such long-term and continuous damage that they couldn't restore the functions. Losing the immune surveillance, the cancer cells were bound to invade and metastasize widely to all of the visceral organs in the whole body.

The real effect of this case was that the treatment killed off tumor cells but damaged the body. It didn't turn out as it should be. In fact, the treatments failed to prevent carcinomatous metastases, essentially damage the function of immunologic and defensive system of the host, attack the ability of the body resistance and promote the invasion and dissemination of cancer cells.

Six months after the operation, metastatic carcinoma of bone appeared. Eight months after the operation, metastatic carcinoma of liver appeared. The radiotherapy and chemotherapy failed to prevent the progression of this disease. How to evaluate the therapeutic effectiveness that the radiotherapy and chemotherapy had on the patient? What kind of role and status did those treatments play and have?

Case 23 Patient Chen ××, male, Thirty-four, counterman, Wuhan, patient history number: 430849

This patient had suffered from the repetitious and irritative dry cough without phlegm for three years. Then this disease was treated as bronchitis. In January 1997, X-ray film of the chest showed large compact shadows in the right upper lung. CT examination reported that there was a compact shadow about the size of 6cm×9cm in the right upper lung. And there was another sarcoidosis behind it about the size of 1.2cm×1.5cm. The sarcoidosis was the central type and had multiple metastases in the lung. On January 11, 1997, the patient underwent the exploratory thoracotomy. In the operation, it could be easily seen that the nidi had widely infiltrated and couldn't be cut off. The tissue slice showed it as the poorly differentiated adenocarcinoma in the right upper lung. Then the chest was closed. In February, March, April and May 1997, the patient accepted postoperative chemotherapies with the drugs of DDP and ADM for one course a month. On July 14, 1997, scanning reexamination showed the enlargement of lump in the right lung. Because the patient suffered from the headache for one week and felt dizzy. The CT scanning of brain showed the brain metastases. Then on July 22, 1997 and July 27, the patient successively underwent the r-scalpel operation for two times. The headache was eased and then disappeared. And on July 13, 1977, the patient came to the anti-cancer coordination group for outpatient treatment, adopting the drugs of XZ-C series. After taking the medicine, the condition of illness was stable. The patient regained a high spirit, a good appetite. The headache and vomit disappeared. The patient walked and talked as the normal people. Three months (one course) after taking the Wuhan Chinese herbal anticancer medicine of XZ-C series, the condition of illness had an obvious improvement. The patient had a rosy cheek, regained the physical strength and walked as the normal people. There was no cough or any kind of discomfort. The breathing sound of right lung faded out. Afterwards the patient accepted the chemotherapy in another hospital, continuously increasing the dose for reinforced chemotherapies. The white blood cell count (WBC) dropped to 300, which was an extremely low value. The immunologic function crocked up.

Analysis: This patient underwent the exploratory thoracotomy for the cancer of right lung. The nidi couldn't be cut off. Then the patient accepted the continuous reinforced chemotherapies. The cancer cells metastasized to the brain. After the r-scalpel operation, the headache disappeared and obtained satisfactory effects. With the immunoregulation treatment of XZ-C series, the general conditions of this patient were getting better obviously and the symptoms improved. But the continuous reinforced chemotherapies resulted in the failure of immunologic function.

11

Review and Prospect of Treatment of Oncology Surgery

- *The achievement of surgical resection of the tumor in the 20th century*
- *21st century surgical goal should be prevention and treatment research for cancer recurrence and metastasis after surgery radical resection*
- *The design of tumor radical surgery should be further studied and perfected*
- *The molecular biology basic research and clinical basic research of metastasis should be strengthened after the radical resection*
- *To prevent cancer recurrence and metastasis should be done from the surgery*

Surgical operation is a definite and effective cure for malignant tumor therapy. Even though today's cancer treatment has developed to the multi-discipline and multimodality treatment, surgical operation is still one of the most central and common means for malignant tumor therapy, and makes itself an integral part of multi-discipline and multimodality treatment.

In the 18th century, therapists held that the early cancer was a local disease, which could be cured by surgical treatment. In 1881, Bill-roth first carried out the surgical removal of tumor — subtotal gastrectomy. In 1890, Halsted actualized the radical resection of breast. He first elucidated the principle of en bloc resection, which meant resections of lymphatic vessel and lymph node in the chosen zone of primary tumor. This resection laid a good foundation for most modern surgical operations of tumors. The surgical technique of tumor resection has been developing along with surgery. After the middle of the 20th century, it gradually developed into an independent subject — tumor surgery. Since the 1950s, due to the improvement and development of surgical technique, preoperative (postoperative) care and operative supporting measures, such as blood transfusion, anesthesia, aseptic technique and antibiotics, the surgical risk, complications and fatality rate have reduced greatly; the range of tumor surgical technique tends to expand; a series of super radical operations arise, such as expansive radical mastectomy. But many years' practice proves that expanding the range of surgical resection cannot improve the survival time without tumor and total survival time of most tumors, such as lung cancer, liver cancer and pancreatic cancer.

Since the 1970s, people's understanding of tumor biology has changed a lot. At present, people hold that most tumors are not local diseases and may have been systemic diseases since the clinical examination. The hematogenous spread is common. When finally diagnosed, many patients may have suffered from micro-metastases. Whether obvious metastases have happened since the clinical examination, depends upon biological characteristics of tumor cells and interactions between tumors and hosts. Neither the more extensive regional surgery nor the share of surgery and radiotherapy can affect metastases.

1. Great Achievements in Surgical Removal of Tumor in 20th Century

In the 20th century, great achievements mainly focus on researching various methods of tumor surgical resections, operation procedures, preoperative (postoperative) care and cleaning range of lymph nodes; studying, understanding and getting familiar with regional anatomy and pathophysiology of bearing cancer organs, such as resection technique and organ reconstruction technique of liver cancer, pancreatic cancer, stomach cancer, esophageal cancer, colorectal cancer, lung cancer, breast cancer, cervical cancer, brain cancer and so on; taking measures to raise resection rate, reduce complications, lower operative mortality rate and improve perioperative care. In terms of esophageal cancer surgery, how to raise the resection rate? How to reduce anastomotic leakage? How to improve Esophagogastrostomy upon (down) Aortic Arch? How to carry out the cervical anastomosis? How to improve anastomose technique, such as scarf-type anastomosis? And in the case of liver cancer, how to perform regular or irregular hepatectomy? How to conduct (expanding) lobectomy of liver? How to carry out combined segmentum hepatis resection, second resection of intrahepatic recurrent cancer after resection, and liver cancer resection of special regions? How to retain residual liver functions? For the breast cancer, how to perform radical or super radical operation? Then how to conduct conservative operation procedures? In the case of stomach cancer, how to carry out D2 and D3 operations? How many groups of lymph nodes are needed to clear? For the operation procedure of rectal cancer, select Mile or Dixon procedure? Retain anus or not? Use anastomat or not? In terms of pancreatic cancer, select Whipple or Child procedure? How to conduct anastomose procedure of gall bladder and bowel? How to perform the resection of hepatic hilar cholangiocarcinoma? For the lung cancer, how to carry out the resection of pulmonary segments, lung lobes or the whole lung? In conclusion, researches are about how to resect the tumor en bloc and completely? How to increase operative resection rate? How to reduce or avoid complications? How to lower operative mortality rate? And how to help patients recover? By the 1990s, cancer resections of esophagus, stomach, bowel, liver, gall bladder, pancreas, lung, mammary gland and thyroid gland fully pass the test. All the operative routine techniques are already mature. Operative mortality rates have dropped to a very low level. Operations are basically safe. Many cancer radical operations have been widely diffused among county hospitals and basic hospitals. But how to prevent recurrence and metastasis has not yet generally attracted people's attention.

In some large hospitals, doctors have perceived that though operations are performed very thoroughly and canonically, postoperative recurrence and metastasis in the short (long) term still puzzle some specialists. Then in the 1990s, some experts have followed suit, announcing the study that disposes cast-off cells caused by operative wound. Chen Junqing in Shenyang has spent over ten years on researching and processing cast-off cells of stomach cancer, finally making brilliant achievements. The study conducted by South Hospital, which heats, washes and processes cast-off cells after the operation of rectum cancer, has got satisfactory efficacy. Yang Chuanyong at Tongji Hospital has always been devoting himself to exploring the pharmacokinetics of intraperitoneal chemotherapy of hepatic portal venous blood. At present, the technique of surgical excision of the tumor is basically successful, which is an honorable achievement in the 20th century. But these difficulties that cancer patients suffer from postoperative recurrences and metastases with no good countermeasure, and frequently come back to the clinic for further consultation, still bother vast numbers of medical workers.

2. The Objectives of Surgery in 21st Century Should Be the Study on Prevention and Control of Recurrence and Metastasis after Radical Operation of Carcinoma

In 1985, the writer himself made follow-up to more than 3,000 patients who had accepted surgical radical excisions of tumors. The results show that 2~3 years after the operation, most patients suffer from recurrences or metastases. While some patients even bear it after six months, less than a year or just over one year. These patients do not always come back to the previous surgery physician for further consultation but go to Tumor Hospital or Tumor Department for medical treatment. Once recurrences appear, however, only a few patients can accept the second operation. But most patients cannot receive effective therapies and soon pass away. It has made the writer more aware that though the operation at that time was successful and standard, the long-term follow-up result is dissatisfactory. That is, the late result is a failure (Certainly tens of patients can survive for 10, 20 or 30 years after the operation, but it is only a very few cases.). Therefore, the study must be done to prevent postoperative recurrence and metastasis. Follow-up results present an important problem that postoperative recurrence or metastasis is the key factor for long-term postoperative effectiveness. While researching method and measure of preventing postoperative recurrence or metastasis plays the key role in improving long-term effectiveness and lengthening survival time. Therefore, the clinical fundamental research must be done for preventing cancer recurrence and metastasis. If no breakthrough in the field of fundamental research, it will be hard to improve clinical effectiveness. Then the writer as well as his colleagues has established the Institute of Experimental Surgery, where they have carried out experimental tumor research, implemented transplantation of cancer cells to animals, constructed tumor animals' models. They have also developed a series of experimental tumor researches: ① Explore mechanism and rule of cancer recurrence and metastasis; ② Probe into the relationship between tumor and immunity, and that between tumor and immune organ; ③ Research into the method of arresting progressive atrophy of immune organs with the growth of tumor and the way of immunologic reconstitution; ④ Seek effective measures to adjust and control cancer invasion, recurrence and metastasis; ⑤ Conduct inhibition rates experiments of tumor-bearing animals to respectively filter 200 literature-approved traditional Chinese medicines which are commonly used for anti-cancer; ⑥ Carry out experimental researches to seek new drugs from natural drugs with resistances to cancer, recurrence and metastasis.

The writer has gone through a complete review of almost 60 year practical cases of clinical treatment and also made the follow-up. Then he analyzes and rethinks the lessons of success and failure, from which he comes to understand a truth. That is, conquering cancer needs to break with the conventional ideas and update the thought; conduct investigations, researches and analyses with patients; carry out self-reflection and self-evaluation. Renew ideas, innovate methods, look for an opening in urgent problems of tumor researches and weak links of modern medicine. The writer has also realized that techniques of surgical resections of tumors in the 20th century have made brilliant achievements. The next researching objective and task of surgeons are not only to have further studies on seeking for greater perfection of radical operation, but also to prevent postoperative recurrence and metastasis. Experiments and clinical researches on preventing recurrence and metastasis after cancer radical operation should be done to further improve postoperative long-term effectiveness. Because the operation is just a regional treatment, if the tumor is limited in a certain visceral organ, the surgical effect may be very good; but if the tumor is not just limited in this visceral organ but has invaded the serosa outside the organ, no matter how thorough the operation is, the possibility of recurrence and metastasis is still in existence. Especially for stomach cancer and rectum cancer, though lymph nodes are cleared completely, many cancer cells still remain in venous blood vessels. A lot of research materials have identified that clearance of lymph nodes is only to prevent lymphatic metastasis but that is just one side. The involved lymph nodes should be cleared, but excising lymph nodes cannot prevent hematogenous metastasis. Therefore, hepatic metastases rates in the short/long term are both high after operations of stomach cancer and intestinal cancer. At present, surgical excision of the tumor as well as regional lymphatic vessels and lymph nodes cannot prevent hematogenous metastasis and spread, implantation and dissemination of cast-off cells. Consequently, the next objective of tumor surgeons' research work should focus on experiments and clinical researches for preventing cancer recurrence and metastasis after radical operation. That is, in the early 20th century, researchers should make great achievements on studies of preventing cancer recurrence and metastasis. If postoperative recurrence and metastasis cannot be solved, short/long-term effectiveness of surgical cancer treatment will fail to get satisfactory result.

3.   Design of Surgical Radical Operation of Tumor to be Further Studied and Perfected

Since recurrence and metastasis happens after the radical operation, it is necessary to analyze whether the radical operation itself has connection with postoperative recurrence and metastasis, and carry out retrospective analysis and reflection. Among the present radical operations, some have been used for over 100 years, such as the radical operation of breast cancer. Over a century, thousands of cancer patients have accepted different kinds of radical operations, the majority of which have got satisfied short-term effectiveness. But long-term recurrence and metastasis rates are still very high. As the name implies, "radical cure" means thorough or eradicating treatment; but if it is "radical operation", why the purpose of radical cure fails to achieve and the recurrence still happens? Now that lymph nodes have been cleared, why the metastasis still appears? The question is whether those recurrences and metastases are due to cast-off cells left by operation or operative techniques, related to procedure design, concept foundation of operative design or not entirely consistent with the present known Biological characteristics and biological behaviors of cancer cells. The present radical operation refers to the en bloc resection of primary tumor and regional lymph nodes. Logically, it is not the radical cure, and cannot approach the purpose of radical cure.

That is because the malignant tumor has four routes of metastasis, which are lymphatic channel metastasis, hematogenous metastasis, implantation metastasis and direct spreading. While the surgical operation just completely clears lymph nodes and radically cures the route of lymphatic channel metastasis, it has no specific technical measure to prevent hematogenous metastasis, and also do nothing to bring forward definite and effective countermeasures to implantation of cast-off cancer cells as well as implantation and dissemination of chest and peritoneal cavity. Lymph nodes having been thoroughly cleared off cannot prevent hematogenous metastasis, and moreover, only the clearance of lymph nodes can't prevent peritoneal implantation and dissemination of peritoneal cavity by cast-off cancer cells, either. Surgical operation belongs to a regional treatment. Experts in tumor surgery hold that cancer develops in a local area of the body, invades the surrounding tissues and metastasizes to other areas through lymphatic vessels, etc. Accordingly, the main point of treatment is often put on the local area, controlling local growth and diffusion, especially lymph nodes metastasis, such as the clearance of lymph nodes. For years surgical treatment has been updating on the operation method and type, but its long-term effectiveness — 5-year survival rate still has no obvious improvement. The postoperative recurrence and metastasis seriously threaten patients' postoperative survival. Therefore, the present radical operation is just a relative one, which is on a quote. Young doctors should know that the present type design still has weak links, which need the further experimental and clinical studies to explore new techniques and methods to definitely and effectively prevent routes of metastases. Accordingly, in recent years the writer's laboratory has always been doing experimental exploration in this respect, such as experimental study of free-tumor technique in radical operation (Fig. 1), free-tumor technique study in radical operation of cancer-bearing animal models, counting of intraoperative cast-off cancer cells as well as detection and counting of cancer cells in venous angioma, experimental observation of dyeing tracking of gastric lymph nodes. Preventing postoperative cancer metastasis and recurrence must be started from the radical operation.

In order to study why cancer cells can dissociate and cast off from the tumor body, cast-off cancer cells still have the vitality and can implant to other areas, the writer's laboratory use electronic microscope to observe and study cancer cells' ultrastructural organization of cancer-bearing animal models (Fig. 2, 3).

Authors: Xu Ze (China) ; Xu Jie(China) ; Bin Wu(America)

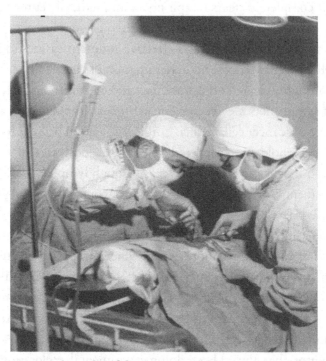

Fig. 1 Experimental study of free-tumor technique in radical operation

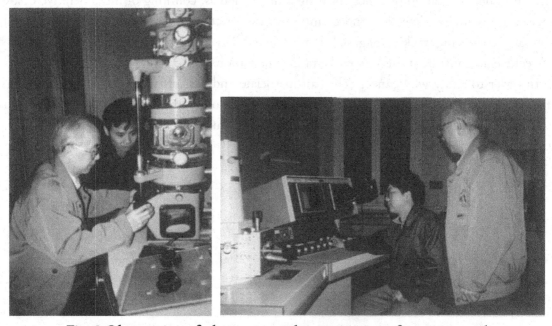

**Fig. 2 Observation of ultrastructural organization of experimental
model's cancer cells with electronic microscope**

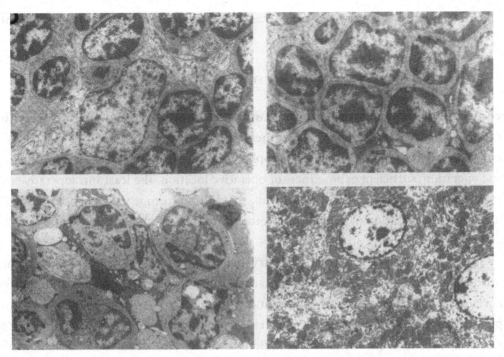

Fig. 3 Ultrastructural organization of hepatic cancer cells of cancer-bearing mouse H$_{22}$

4. **Strengthening Fundamental and Clinical Study on Molecular Biology of Radical Operation of Recurrence and Metastasis after Operation**

Inhibiting angiogenesis factors to induce the formation of blood vessels and preventing endothelial cells to construct new blood vessels are both new ways to explore preventions from recurrence and metastasis. In the experimental study of inhibiting actions of ethyl acetate extractives (TG) of traditional Chinese medicine — Common Threewingnut Root with different dosages on new blood vessels of transplanted tumor of mice peritoneum, the writer's laboratory observe influences of TG on the form and number of new-born micro-vessels in and around transplanted tumor of mice peritoneum, and on the diameter and flow rate of tumor arterioles and venules. They have made the preliminary confirmation that TG has certain inhibiting actions on new-born blood vessels of metastatic carcinoma focus and has been taken on clinical trials.

Study of preventing postoperative recurrence and metastasis of cancers must base on establishing animal models of recurrence and metastasis, and also proceed on levels of Molecular Biology and Gene. In the past decade and more, due to the rapid development of Molecular Biology, experts have found that the generation, progress, invasion, metastasis and recurrence of tumor are all in connection with cancer genes, cancer suppressor genes, metastatic genes and suppressor metastatic genes. To research related genes and seek control methods to prevent recurrence and metastasis as well as clinical measures of preventing recurrence, such as biological therapy, gene therapy, biological reaction control agent therapy, may be an important research aim in the future. In the 21st century, gene therapy will provide new efficient way for tumor therapy, and Molecular Biological Immunology will also stimulate the development of tumor therapy.

5. **Prevention of Recurrence and Metastasis after Operation Should Be Established in Operation**

(1) **Surgical techniques of cancer surgery**

Free-tumor technique is vitally important, which should prevent operation techniques from causing or actuating hematogenous metastasis of cancer cells.

Surgical principles of general surgery also applies to tumor surgery, such as operation techniques of aseptic operation, sufficient exposedness of operative location, the least intraoperative damage of normal tissues for the early-stage healing, etc. In addition, tumor surgery should take note of preventing the dissemination of cancer cells in the operation, in which the free-tumor technique is vitally important.

Ever since the end of the nineteenth century, people have realized that operation techniques may cause or actuate the dissemination of cancer cells. Therefore, the free-tumor technique of tumor surgery has been attracting more and more attention in recent years. For instance, intraoperative procedures of preserved skin, extrusion and anatomy can directly lead to the dissemination of tumor cells, stimulate formations of tumor embolism and metastasis which are near to or far away from blood vessels and lymphatic vessel. And tumor cells cast off and pollute surgical wounds, which results in local implantation recurrence, etc. Along with the development of Cell Pathology and inspection technology of tumor cells in blood stream, the phenomenon of tumor dissemination has been confirmed in clinical trials and animal experiments. For example, active cancer cells and cancer tissue masses can be found in vessel douche and surgical wounds douche of tumor operative specimen; cancer cells can be easier found in the output venous blood flow of tumor during the operation. Therefore, it is important that in the operation surgeons should first ligate and cut off output vena of tumor.

It should be noted in surgical operation that all the techniques are favorable toward preventing cancer cells' metastases. Do not stimulate or increase chances of cancer cells' metastases to cause iatrogenic metastasis and dissemination. For the surgical resection of tumor, all the operations must stress and observe free-tumor concept and technique, no matter big or small. Surgeons should give equal emphasis on free-tumor concept and aseptic concept, free-tumor technique and aseptic technique. The free-tumor technique is even stricter than aseptic technique. The surgical knife, scissors, needle and thread in the surgical operation, even every procedure is possible to cause metastasis of cancer cells. Such a possibility may increase with excessive extrusion, needle punching through the skin, knife cutting and other negative operative procedures by surgeons on tumor body or tissues. At present, applied molecular biology or immunohistochemistry method has proved that the operation technique itself can cause iatrogenic implantations, diffusions and metastases of cancer cells. Cancer cells can be found in surrounding blood circulations when many patients are undergoing the surgical operation; or cancer cells convert from the preoperative negative result to the postoperative positive result. The above evidences indicate that operation techniques are possible to induce the diffusion of cancer cells. It also suggests that some patients' postoperative recurrence and metastasis may be caused by improper operation techniques, such as the incision implantation.

Therefore, preventing postoperative recurrence and metastasis must start out from all the techniques in the surgical operation.

The route and type of tumor dissemination vary according to different pathologic types of tumor. Whether or not the metastasis can come into being is also related to the body's immune state. Consequently during the therapeutic process, the modern tumor surgeons should both prevent tumor dissemination and be careful to maintain the body's resistibility or immunity.

(2) **Prevention from the dissemination of cancer cells**

It is well-known but always overlooked that tumor's localized examination and operation techniques should be gentle and skillful to prevent the dissemination of cancer cells. Therefore, the following points should be noted: ① Preoperative tumor palpation should be gentle, and the number of times ought to be minimized. ② Preserved skin for operation should be gentle and skillful, or more cancer cells will invade small veins by the over friction. ③ operation techniques should be gentle and skillful, incision must be sufficient to expose, dissect and resect. Avoid pressing the tumor. ④ Adopt sharp dissection (dissecting knife or scissor); Strictly avoid blunt dissection to reduce dissemination. ⑤ Deal with the output vein before the artery. ⑥ Dispose the farther lymph nodes before the nearby lymph nodes to resect them wholly with the tumor.

(3) **Prevention from the implantation of cancer cells**

Cast-off cancer cells easily implant and grow on the traumatic tissue wounds, so: ① Use the gauze pad to protect cutting shoulder and wound surface. ② if the tumor is unwittingly incised or cracks, it should be covered and bound up with gauze pads. Replace timely polluted gloves and surgical instruments. ③ Adequate excision extent, involving enough normal tissues around the pathological changes. ④ Avoid the blood out-flowing from polluted wounds when anatomizing tissues near the tumor. Therefore, when two blood vessel forceps are used to clamp blood vessels, they should stick close to each other. Ligate immediately after being cut off. Replace timely gauze pads that are contaminated with blood.

Postoperative local recurrence (cover about 10%) of colon and rectum cancers often occurs in anastomotic stoma, incision of abdominal wall or outside of intestinal wall. This kind of recurrence is usually caused by the implantation of cancer cells. In recent years, a strip of cloth is used to ligate intestinal canals belonging to the upper and lower segment of tumor before the excision of intestinal loop, in order to stop cast-off cancer cells from continuing to diffuse along the intestinal cavity in the surgical operation. Use 1:500 corrosive sublimate or fluorouracil solution to douche intestinal cavities of both ends before the anastomosis, which can obviously improve the long-term effectiveness and may be relevant to the before-mentioned reduction of recurrence.

After all, to review significant achievements of 20-century techniques of surgical tumor excision; to preview glary prospects of 21-century tumor surgery study of prevention from recurrence and metastasis. In the coming period, the highlight of anti-cancer work should be anti-invasion, anti-metastasis and anti-recurrence. Anti-recurrence is the key of operative effectiveness; and anti-metastasis is the core question of cancer treatment. Cancer invasion and

Authors: Xu Ze (China) ; Xu Jie(China) ; Bin Wu(America)

metastasis depend on specific potentials of two factors: biological characteristics of tumor cell itself and the host's influence on its restraining factors. To keep a balance is to control; to lose a balance is to progress.

The Advocacy for the Formation and Development of Traditional Therapies

```
┌─────────────────────────────────────────────────────┐
│            In the last two centuries the treatment of │
│            malignant tumors appeared twice leaps      │
└─────────────────────────────────────────────────────┘
                          ↓
┌─────────────────────────────────────────────────────┐
│            The first time was that in 1989 Halsted    │
│            proposed the concept of radical surgery     │
└─────────────────────────────────────────────────────┘
                          ↓
┌─────────────────────────────────────────────────────┐
│            The second was that in the 1970s Fish integrated │
│            chemotherapy with radical surgery (adjuvant │
│            chemotherapy or neoadjuvant chemotherapy)   │
└─────────────────────────────────────────────────────┘
                          ↓
┌─────────────────────────────────────────────────────┐
│     Since then the treatment of malignant tumors were wandering, │
│     the death rate of malignant tumor death is still the first │
└─────────────────────────────────────────────────────┘
```

Radical surgery	chemotherapy with radical surgery (adjuvant chemotherapy or neoadjuvant chemotherapy)
Extended radical surgery Super radical surgery	Target of Radiotherapy and chemotherapy is to kill cancer cells and at the same time kill proliferating cells and immune cells
Modified radical surgery	Didn't improve the efficacy, and toxic side effects happened and it reduce immunity
Professor Xu Ze proposed the following four points of reform and development	Professor Xu Ze proposed the following six points of reform and development

The design of radical resection should be further studied and perfected

Point out that cure should be regulated rather than single kill

put forward that Tumor-free technology Surgical Oncology is extremely important

A comprehensive treatment concept should be established for both host and cancer cells

Prevent cancer cells spread from running blood during surgery Spread

Pointed out that chemotherapy needs further research and improvement of immunotherapy

Preventing implanting of exfoliated cancer cells during surgery

Questioning the route of administration of systemic intravenous chemotherapy for solid tumors

Initiative of systemic intravenous chemotherapy for solid tumors as target organ intravascular chemotherapy

Initiative chemotherapy for postoperative adjuvant chemotherapy for intraperitoneal venous catheterization

III. The Brief and Easy-Reading Epitome of Walking out the New Way of Conquering Cancer

A series of Anti-cancer, anti-cancer metastasis research, scientific and technological innovation, scientific research results series
Technological innovation
Scientific research results

Walked out of a new road to overcome cancer
——XX-C immunomodulation anticancer treatment has been initially formed
——In the past 60 years, a new road to overcome cancer has been walked out

(the short reading version)

Foreword

Why did I take the title of the book as: "Walking out of a new road to overcome cancer", the title of the book is due to the guidance and inspiration from several experts, scholars, seniors, and teachers.

On July 2, 2001, Academician Wu Wei mentioned in his letter: "**The overall impression is: the mode from clinical to experimental and back from experimental to clinical is very good, the road of combining Chinese medicine with Western medicine is also very correct, I sincerely wish you keep moving forward and walk out of a new path to overcome cancer.**"

On February 22, 2006, Academician Tang Yu mentioned in his letter: "... **Chinese medicine and Chinese medication and biological therapy are the two most promising ways to resist metastasis, especially Chinese medication. I hope that you will walk out of the anti-metastasis road with Chinese characteristics.**"

On March 22, 2006, Academician Liu Yunyi mentioned in his letter: "...**I agree with your concept and thinking about cancer in your book... I hope that you can make a breakthrough contribution to traditional Chinese medicine again to make the benefits for the majority of patients and to make the traditional Chinese medicine be further developed, and to make my medical career reach a world status.**"

On January 9, 2006, Academician Wu Xianzhong mentioned in his letter: "...**the tumor is a difficult bone or the tumor is a hard bone, but it should continue to work on or it should continue to be continued. Fortunately, everyone is very objective, as long as it is effective, whether it is treating the tumor or the body, or reducing the reaction of the Chemotherapy or radiotherapy, the support will be given**. In the letter of April 10, 2012, "**We think that the road you have traveled is very special or very distinctive**. On the application formulation and the methods of taking or using and the drug combinations of the traditional Chinese medication, XZ-C drugs series have all innovated and developed and formed their own patents. **This road should continue to go or walk on.**"

Thanks for their guidance, guidance, and assistance in our research work, research thinking, research direction, research routes, research goals, and research methods. Thanks for their guidance, leading, and assistance in our research work, research thinking, research direction, research routes, research goals, and research methods. Our research work has been working in the direction of these guidance. I would like to express my gratitude to the academicians Wu Hao, Tang Wei, Wu Xianzhong and Liu Yunyi.

In the past 33 years (1985-present), cancer research has achieved a series of scientific and technological innovations and scientific research achievements in animal experimental research, clinical basic research and clinical verification. After more than 30 years of hard work, XZ-C immune regulation and control Anti-cancer treatment has been formed. In the past more than 30 years, a new road to conquer cancer has been taken out.

In the past 20 years, this series of experimental and clinical research work has received warm support and cordial guidance from Professor **Qiu Fazu**, who was the internationally renowned surgeon and the Master of the general surgery in China. In 1990, when the author submitted the "Eighth Five-Year Plan" key scientific and technological research project to the State Science and Technology Commission (the application of further exploring the anti-cancer and anti-metastasis experimental and clinical studies of cancer and anti-cancer Chinese herbal medicine for precancerous lesions of liver cancer and gastrointestinal cancer), Academician **Qiu Fazu** said in an expert opinion: "**It is a very important topic to study cancer metastasis and how to prevent metastasis. It is feasible to explore clinical prevention methods through experimental research and it is beneficial to people's work**." Under the meditate and guidance of the rigorous and scientific style of study of my teacher and Academican Qiu Fazu, we have completed the above projects, and I would like to thank you.

Scientific research must have nutritional feeding of the literature. In 1986, we just established an experimental surgical animal laboratory to make an animal model of cancer metastasis and conduct experimental research. We saw Professor Gao Jin's book "**Invasion and Metastasis of Cancer - Basic Research and Clinical Medicine**", and saw the monograph of Academician Tang Wei, "**Basic and Clinical Metastasis and Recurrence of Liver Cancer**". Theories in the two books make us suddenly see the light, or be clear. It also encourages and promotes our experimental work and clinical validation work from another aspect. Professor Tang Wei proposed in his monograph: "**The next important goal of primary liver cancer research - prevention and treatment of recurrence and metastasis**", and said: "**metastasis and recurrence have become a bottleneck to further improve the survival rate of liver cancer, and is one of the most important difficulties in combating cancer.**" **These theoretical documents have given us the wisdom and courage to update our thinking and be brave in innovation, and have also strengthened the confidence and determination of our experimental team.** Here I would like to express my gratitude to Academician Tang Wei and Professor Gao Jin.

In the past 7 years, we have used more than 6,000 tumor-bearing animal models to explore one basic problem after another. The screening of 200 kinds of Chinese herbal medicines in the tumor-bearing animal model in vivo was carried out by several graduate students. Master Zhu Siping, Dr. Zou Shaomin, Master Li Zhengxun, Master of Liu Wei, etc., they carried out and completed a lot of hard and meticulous experimental work, take great pains, day and night, contributed to the development of experimental oncology medicine career for cancer prevention and anti-cancer. In hereI sincerely thank you all.

Contents

(1)   the concept of cancer treatment 221

(2)   the cause and pathogenesis of cancer 222

(3)   Theoretical basis and experimental basis for cancer treatment 223

(4)   principles of cancer treatment 224

(5)   Cancer treatment mode 225

(6)   Principles of cancer metastasis treatment 226

(7)   The main features of the new concept of cancer treatment - control transfer 227

(8)   New concept of cancer metastasis treatment 228

(9)   A new concept of cancer metastasis treatment - the third form of cancer in the
human body is the cancer cell group on the way to transfer 229

(10)   A new concept of cancer metastasis treatment - "two points and one line theory" 231

(11)   "Three Steps" for Cancer Metastasis Treatment 233

(12)   A new concept of cancer metastasis treatment - opening up the third field of
human anti-cancer metastasis treatmen 236

(13)   Experimental screening of XZ-C immunomodulatory anticancer Chinese medicine 238

(14)   Cancer treatment methods and drugs - A, B, C, D 239

(15)   Immunomodulatory pharmacology of XZ-C immunomodulation anticancer
Chinese medication 245

(16)   The indications and application ranges of XZ-C$_{1-10}$ immunomodulation Chinese
medication anti-cancer metastasis and recurrence clinical applications 246

(17)   Study on XZ-C immunomodulation of anticancer traditional Chinese medicine 247

(18)   XZ-C immunomodulation cancer treatment of cancer cases list 248

(19)   The formation of the theoretical system of XZ-C treatment 251

(20)   The book proposed XZ-C new concept cancer therapy, which was analyzed and
compared with traditional therapy, and analyzed by table: 252

(一)1

the concept of cancer treatment

The new model believes that healing should be regulated and controlled rather than killed

[Summary]

1. The traditional concept holds that cancer is the continuous division and proliferation of cancer cells, and its therapeutic goal must be to kill cancer cells. Therefore, the traditional therapeutic concept of cancer is based on the killing of cancer cells.
2. the new model of cancer believes that: cure should be through regulation and control rather than killing, the final step in curing cancer is to mobilize the reproduction of host control instead of destroying the last cancer cells. Why? Because of killing only can kill canner cells during those days of using the medications, it can't be done once and for all; after that, it still divides proliferation, recurrence, progression. Mitigation is only a temporary phenomenon.

（二）2

the cause and pathogenesis of cancer

XU proposes that thymus atrophy and immune dysfunction may be one of the causes and pathogenesis of cancer.

[Summary]

This book first proposed in the international community "one of the causes and pathogenesis of cancer may be thymus atrophy and immune function is low." After investigation: this is the first time in the world.

Our laboratory found from the experimental results that the thymus of the cancer-bearing mice showed progressive atrophy, the volume was reduced, the cell proliferation was blocked, and the mature cells were reduced. By the end of the tumor, the thymus is extremely atrophied and the texture becomes hard. It may be atrophy of the thymus, impaired central immune function, low immune function, decreased immune surveillance and immune escape.

(三)3

Theoretical basis and experimental basis for cancer treatment

XZ proposed: the theoretical basis and experimental basis for the treatment of "protecting the thymus and lifting the immune function"

[Summary]

In this book, it was firstly proposed that the theoretical basis and experimental basis of the therapeutic principle of XZ-C immunomodulation therapy--protecting Thymus and increasing the immune function (protecting the thymus, increasing immunity) and protecting the marrow and hematopoietic for blood (protecting bone marrow stem cells). This is the first time internationally presented.

Because the above experimental research finds new inspiration, its treatment principle must be to prevent progressive atrophy of the thymus, promote thymic hyperplasia, protect bone marrow hematopoietic function, improve immune surveillance, and control immune escape of malignant cells.

Therefore, its treatment should be "protecting Thymus and increasing immune function " to protect the thymus and boost immunity. It is the theoretical basis and experimental basis for the "protection of Thymus and increase or enhancement of immune function t" of XZ-C immunomodulation therapy.

（四）4

principles of cancer treatment

——XZ proposes to establish a comprehensive treatment concept

[Summary]

This book first puts forward <<the goal or target of cancer treatment in the world must establish a comprehensive treatment concept for both tumor and host>>. At present, chemotherapy and chemotherapy in the hospitals at home and abroad is only and simple to kill cancer cells. We think this is one-sided treatment concept which is not only does not protect the patient's immunity, but also kills the host's immune cells and bone marrow hematopoietic cells in large numbers, resulting in there is more chemotherapy and there is the lower the immunity function so that there is the cancer matastasis while there is chemotherapy. We advocate that all hospitals around the world should establish a comprehensive treatment concept for both radiotherapy and chemotherapy and reform the current status of the one-sided treatment concept. No one has mentioned the concept of "comprehensive treatment" or "one-sided treatment" in the past. This concept was first proposed internationally.

（五）5

Cancer treatment mode

——XZ proposes to establish a multidisciplinary comprehensive treatment plan

Summary]

This book first proposes <<the initiative to establish a multidisciplinary comprehensive treatment plan.>> At present, hospitals at home and abroad are mainly focusing on radiotherapy and chemotherapy. At present, the current status of comprehensive treatment in various provinces in China is based on traditional three major treatments. The results of comprehensive treatment still do not prevent recurrence and metastasis. As for biological treatment and immunotherapy, Differentiation and induction therapy, combination of Chinese and Western medicine, and immunomodulation therapy were not included in the treatment plan of oncologists.

We propose to propose:

The whole process of treatment is the main axis: surgery-based + biological treatment, immune regulation treatment, integrated Chinese and Western medicine treatment, XZ-C immunomodulation treatment......

Short-course treatment is the auxiliary axis: mainly for radiotherapy and chemotherapy. It is not a long course of treatment. It should not be excessive. It should change the current status of over-treatment of some hospitals.

This new concept of full-course treatment and short-course treatment was first proposed internationally.

（六）6

Principles of cancer metastasis treatment

—— the key of cancer treatment is anti-metastasis

[Summary]

This book proposes that the key to cancer research is anti-metastasis, the basic principle of cancer treatment is anti-metastasis, the main feature of the new concept of cancer treatment, is namely control metastasis.

Metastasis is the leading cause of cancer death, so metastasis is the key to cancer treatment.

The main cause of such high mortality is cancer. The original traditional treatment failed to reduce the long-term high mortality rate. The main reason for the failure was the failure to target transfer and control transfer.

Today, the main problem with cancer treatment is how to resist metastasis. If the problem of cancer metastasis cannot be solved, cancer treatment cannot be advanced. Therefore, one of the goals of cancer treatment in the 21st century should be anti-metastasis.

（七）7

The main features of the new concept of cancer treatment - control transfer

XZ believes: Control transfer, protect patient immunity, not simply kill cancer cells

[Summary]

How to control transfer? Killing human cancer cells should rely on two kinds of forces: one is the external force of surgery, radiotherapy, and chemotherapy; the other is the internal strength of the patient's own immunity.

Drugs, surgery, and various treatment techniques are important for the treatment of patients, but the body's own immunity is more important.

Many problems must be resolved by the patient's own strength, because there is a complete anti-cancer system in the human body.

why? Because the main feature of the new concept of cancer treatment is to control the transfer and protect the patient's immunity, instead of simply killing cancer cells.

（八）8

New concept of cancer metastasis treatment

Targets of anti-metastasis should target cancer cells on the way to metastasis

Summary]

This book first published a new theoretical understanding in the world, and proposed a new concept of cancer anti-metastasis treatment: there are three manifestations of cancer in the human body: the first is primary cancer; the second is metastatic cancer; the third It is a group of cancer cells on the way to transfer.

Targets that are resistant to metastasis or "targets" of treatment should target cancer cell populations on the way to metastasis. In fact, the new treatment mode for coagulation, obstruction or interference against the cancer cell group on the way of metastasis and cutting off the metastasis pathway is the key to anti-cancer metastasis. According to the cancer cell transfer pathway, it is to design a new anti-metastatic treatment model for cofferdam obstruction.

why? Because the third manifestation is the metastasis of cancer cells, cancer cell populations and micro-cancer plugs on the way. To design a new anti-metastatic treatment model to aim the Intercepting the cancer cell population on the way to the metastasis , this new doctrine is proposed,

A new concept of cancer metastasis treatment - the third form of cancer in the human body is the cancer cell group on the way to transfer

[Summary]

This book first discovers and proposes a new theory or a new theoretical understanding in the world: it proposes that there are three manifestations of cancer in the human body, and its third form in the human body is the cancer cell group on the way to metastasis.

The main manifestations of cancer in the human body, two different cancer therapeutic concepts, have two different perceptions:

(1) The traditional concept of cancer therapy believes that there are two manifestations:
    The first manifestation - primary cancer;
    The second form of expression - metastatic cancer.
    Traditional cancer therapeutic goals or "targets" are for both forms,
    One is for the first manifestation - primary cancer;
    The second is for the second form of expression - metastatic cancer.

This traditional therapeutic concept has been in use for more than a hundred years, and its therapeutic goals or "targets" are directed at these two manifestations - primary or metastatic. Ignore the cancer cells on the way. It is well known that metastasis is the biological characteristics and biological behavior of malignant tumors. The difference between benign tumors and malignant tumors is that the former does not metastasize and the latter metastasizes, and anti-metastasis is the key to cancer treatment. Without blocking the cancer cells on the way to the metastasis, it is impossible to control the metastasis of cancer cells, and thus it is difficult to obtain the possibility of cancer treatment healing.

Authors: Xu Ze (China) ; Xu Jie(China) ; Bin Wu(America)

(2) Xu Ze (XU ZE) has a new concept of cancer treatment. There are three forms of cancer. There are three manifestations of cancer in the human body:

The first manifestation - primary cancer;

The second form of expression - metastatic cancer;

The third manifestation is the metastasis of cancer cells, cancer cell populations and micro-cancer plugs on the way.

The target or "target" of treatment is also directed at these three manifestations:

One is for the first manifestation - primary cancer;

The second is for the second form of expression - metastatic cancer;

The third is for the third manifestation - the cancer cell group on the way to transfer.

This new concept holds that cancer exists in three forms in the human body. It is relatively complete and comprehensive. It clarifies the dynamic relationship, causality and affiliation between the three, and is a complete concept of cancer treatment. A comprehensive explanation of the whole process of cancer development and how to control the whole process of cancer cell metastasis. This new doctrine will bring the dawn of victory over cancer.

(十) 10

A new concept of cancer metastasis treatment
- "two points and one line theory"

[Summary]

This book first proposes another new theory or new theoretical understanding in the world: the "two points and one line" theory of the whole process of cancer development. It is believed that in the treatment of cancer, the past and present have only recognized and valued two points at home and abroad, ignoring the front line. In fact, the treatment of cancer should not only pay attention to two points, but also pay attention to the front line and cut off the first line, which is the key to anti-cancer metastasis.

What is two points and one line? Two points are the starting point of metastasis, primary cancer; and the end point of metastasis, metastatic cancer. A line of cancer cells between the primary tumor and the metastatic tumor travels long distances to the route of metastasis to the distant organs. (see photo)

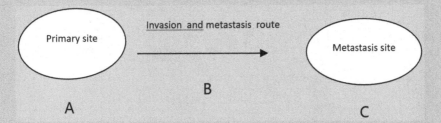

Two-point and one-line diagram of the whole process of cancer cell metastasis

Authors: Xu Ze (China) ; Xu Jie(China) ; Bin Wu(America)

Note: A: primary cancer, metastatic origin; B, route of invasion and metastasis; C, metastatic cancer, metastasis.

Traditional cancer treatment often only pays attention to "two points" but ignores the "first line."

The new concept of XU ZE cancer treatment believes that both "two points" should be emphasized, and the front line should be cut off.

In summary, it can be seen that the new concept of XU ZE cancer treatment not only pays attention to the surgical resection and radiotherapy and chemotherapy of primary and metastatic cancer, but also pays attention to the interception and killing of cancer cells in the process of metastasis. This new theory, called "two points and one line", is of great significance:

In order to Emphasize that anti-transfer it should not only pay attention to "two points", but also pay more attention to "first line." Only by cutting off the cancer cells in the process of metastasis can the cancer treatment effect be improved.

"Three Steps" for Cancer Metastasis Treatment

[Summary]

How to resist transfer? The transfer steps should be understood to make the treatment goals more specific. This book proposes an "eight-step" theory of cancer cell metastasis in order to summarize the extremely complex, dynamic, continuous multi-step, multi-factor cancer cell metastasis process. For scientific design and blocking each transfer step and each break, based on this "eight-step", "three-stage" theory and the molecular mechanism of cancer cell metastasis, the author designed and developed various stages of prevention and treatment measures, called "three-step" of anti-cancer metastasis treatment.

The first step in anti-cancer metastasis is to prevent cancer cells from entering the blood vessels and achieve the goal of "being outside the country".

The second step of anti-cancer metastasis is to activate immune cells, protect thymus tissue function, enhance immunity, protect blood vessels from the marrow, and promote cancer cells that float in the vascular circulation are captured, swallowed, and encircled by the immune cell population.

The third step of anti-cancer metastasis, prevention and treatment goal: to improve the local micro-environmental tissue immunity, make cancer cells difficult to implant, inhibit angiogenesis factors, inhibit the formation of new blood vessels, and suppress countermeasures.

why? The above-mentioned anti-cancer metastasis treatment "three-step" will position the treatment of cancer metastasis in the blood circulation, and the time is located at three different stages, with emphasis on improving host immunity and regulating the local microenvironment.

Anti-cancer metastasis treatment "trilogy, Positioning the space for treating cancer metastasis in the blood circulation, time is positioned at three different stages. The focus is on improving host immunity, which can be summarized as Table 9-1 and Figure 9-1.

Table 9-1 Anti-cancer metastasis treatment "Trilogy"

Metastasis stage of cancer cell	Metastasis process	Prevention and cure countermeasures
Cancer cells invade the pre-circulation phase, the first step of anti-metastasis	Cancer cells are isolated from primary cancer → reduce ECM → adhesion and de-adhesion → exercise → before entering the blood vessel	• anti-adhesion • Anti-degradation • Anti-movement • Anti-matrix metalloproteinase • Block cancer cells outside the blood vessels
Cancer cells in the blood circulation, the transport phase, the second step of anti-metastasis,	Cancer cell populations and tiny cancer plugs drift in the blood circulation and withstand Phagocytosis and endure the capture of immune cells and experience blood shear force impact loss	• Enhance and activate various immune cells and immune factors in the circulation. Raise immune function, the main battlefield for cancer cells on the way to quench • Anti-adhesion • Anti-platelet aggregation • Anti-cancer
Cancer cells escape from the blood circulation and anchor the "target" organ tissue stage, that is, the third step of anti-metastasis	After the cancer cells escape from the blood vessels, the "target" organ tissues are anchored, and new blood vessels are formed to form metastases.	• Inhibition of angiogenic factors • Inhibition of blood vessel formation • Increase immune regulation • Improve local microenvironmental tissue immunity

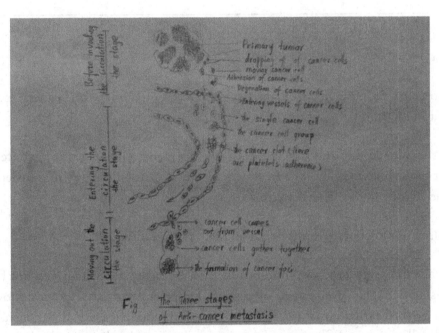

Figure. The three steps of cancer metastasis

（十二）**12**

A new concept of cancer metastasis treatment - opening up the third field of human anti-cancer metastasis treatmen

[Summary]

This book first proposes to open up the third field of human anti-cancer metastasis treatment in the world.

What is the third field of anti-cancer metastasis treatment? All of the third manifestations of cancer in the human body - the treatment of cancer cells on the way to transfer, can be called the third field of anti-cancer treatment.

How to intercept metastatic cancer cells on the way to transfer?

Cancer patients usually have low immune function, especially the cellular immune function is decreasing with the development of tumors. However, many studies have shown that although tumor-bearing hosts may have systemic immunodeficiency, they generally have normal T cell responses. Effective anti-cancer responses can be elicited in both animal and clinical studies. The key is how to break the tumor's inhibition of the immune system and stimulate an effective immune response, especially based on T cells.

How to effectively regulate the host immune function, improve the local immune microenvironment, and facilitate the host anti-cancer effect, is an important and effective measure to prevent postoperative metastasis, recurrence and elimination of residual cancer cells. It is an important part of comprehensive cancer treatment.

The circulatory system has a large number of immune monitoring cells

Cancer cells are engulfed, blocked, captured and swallowed by immune cells in the blood circulation. Therefore, it can be said that blood circulation is the main battlefield for quenching cancer cells on the way to metastasis. Immune cells are the living forces that kill cancer cells.

The circulatory system has a large number of immune monitoring cells, which can kill and phagocytose cancer cells with heterosexual antigens, plus the impact and shear force of blood flow. It is difficult for a single cancer cell to survive. Cancer cells evade the killing of immune cells. It adheres to the inner wall of the blood vessel and adheres to the inner wall of the blood vessel. The endothelial cells in the inner wall of the blood vessel do amoeba movement, and settle in the new organ through the microvascular, and gradually form a new metastatic lesion.

The cancer cells in these metastasis processes are actually the third form of expression in the human body. It is necessary to find a way to respond to the third field of anticancer treatment.

(十三) 13

Experimental screening of XZ-C immunomodulatory anticancer Chinese medicine

[Summary]

XZ-C immunomodulation anticancer Chinese medicine is an experimental study on screening Chinese new anticancer and anti-metastatic drugs from traditional Chinese herbal medicines in our laboratory:

1. In vitro screening test: In vitro culture of cancer cells was used to observe direct damage of cancer cells to cancer cells.
2. in vivo anti-tumor screening experiment: the production of cancer-bearing animal models, the Chinese herbal medicine against cancer-bearing animals in vivo inhibition rate.
3. Experimental results: Among the 200 kinds of Chinese herbal medicines screened by animal experiments in our laboratory, 48 kinds of 48 kinds of Chinese herbal medicines were selected, which had certain inhibitory effects on cancer cells, and the tumor inhibition rate was above 75-95%. This group was screened by animal experiments and eliminated 152 kinds of anti-cancer effects. The main pharmacological effects of XZ-C immunomodulation anti-cancer Chinese medicine are "protection of Thymus and increase of immune " and "protection of blood marrow and hematopoiet

（十四）14

Cancer treatment methods and drugs - A, B, C, D

A. One of the experimental screenings of XZ-C immunomodulatory anticancer Chinese medication

Our laboratory conducted the following experimental studies to screen new anticancer and anti-metastatic drugs from traditional Chinese medications:

(A) The method of in vitro culture of cancer cells was used to screen the cancer suppression rate of Chinese herbal medicines; in vitro screening test: the cancer cells were cultured in vitro to observe the direct damage of the drugs to cancer cells.

In-vitro screening test: in the test tube for culturing cancer cells, biological crude products (500 ug/ml) were separately placed to observe whether they inhibited cancer cells or not. We will take 200 kinds of Chinese herbal medicines that traditional Chinese medicine believes have anti-cancer effects to screen them. Screening experiments were performed in vitro one by one. The toxicity of the drug to the cells was tested by normal fiber cell culture under the same conditions and then compared.

Authors: Xu Ze (China) ; Xu Jie(China) ; Bin Wu(America)

(B) Making tumor-bearing animal models and conducting experimental screening of Chinese herbal medicines for cancer suppression rate in cancer-bearing animals

In vivo anti-cancer screening test, each batch of 240 mice, divided into 8 groups, 30 in each group, the seventh group was a blank control group, the eighth group with 5-FU or CTX as a control group, the whole group of mice Inoculate EAC or S180 or H22 cancer cells. After inoculation for 24 hours, each rat was orally fed with crude drug powder, and the traditional Chinese medicine was fed and screened for a long time. The survival time, toxicity and side effects were observed and calculated, the survival rate was calculated, and the cancer inhibition rate was calculated.

In this way, we conducted a four-year experimental study, and conducted an experimental study on the pathogenesis, metastasis, and recurrence mechanism of tumor-bearing mice for three years, and an experimental study to explore how tumors cause host death. More than 1,000 tumor-bearing animals are used each year. In the model, nearly 6000 tumor-bearing animal models were made in 4 years. After the death of each mouse, the pathological anatomy of the liver, spleen, lung, thymus and kidney was performed. A total of 20,000 slices were taken to explore whether to find out whether There may be carcinogenic micro-pathogens, and microcirculation microscopy was used to observe the microvascular establishment and microcirculation in 100 tumor-bearing mice.

B. Two of the experimental screenings of XZ-C immunomodulatory anticancer Chinese medication

Through experimental research, we have found for the first time in China that TG has a significant effect on inhibiting tumor microvessel formation. It has been used in more than 80 clinical patients for anti-metastasis treatment, and the efficacy is being observed.

Experimental results: Among the 200 kinds of Chinese herbal medicines screened by animal experiments in our laboratory, 48 kinds of Chinese herbal medicines which have certain or even excellent inhibitory effects on cancer cell proliferation were selected, and the tumor inhibition rate was above 75-90%. However, there are also some commonly used traditional Chinese medicines that are generally considered to have anti-cancer effects. After screening for animal tumors in vitro and in vivo, there is no anti-cancer effect, or the effect is very small. In this group, 152 kinds of anti-cancer effects were eliminated by animal experiments.

The 48 kinds of traditional Chinese medicines with good cancer suppression rate were selected by this experiment, and then the optimized combination was repeated to carry out the experiment of cancer suppression rate in cancer. Finally, XZ-C 1-10 immune-regulating anti-cancer Chinese medicines with its own characteristics was developed..

XZ-C1 can significantly inhibit cancer cells, but does not affect normal cells; XZ-C4 can promote thymic hyperplasia and increase immunity; XZ-C8 can protect the marrow from hematopoiesis and protect bone marrow hematopoietic function.

C. Three of the Experimental screening of C and XZ-C immunomodulatory anticancer Chinese medicine ----------Clinical verification

Clinical validation:

On the basis of the success of animal experiments, clinical validation was carried out. That is to establish a tumor specialist clinic and a combination of Chinese and Western medicine for anti-cancer, anti-metastasis and recurrence research, retain the outpatient medical record, establish a regular follow-up observation system, and observe the long-term efficacy.

From experimental research to clinical validation, new problems are discovered during the clinical validation process, and go back to the laboratory for basic research, and again the new experimental results are applied to clinical validation

D. Foutth of the Experimental screening of C and XZ-C immunomodulatory anticancer Chinese medicine ----------Clinical verification

(1) Among the 4277 patients with advanced cancer who were treated with XZ-C$_{1\text{-}10}$ immunomodulatory TCM for more than 3 months, the medical records were recorded in detail. See the table below:

The Observation of curative effect on 4277 cases:
Comprehensive improved the quality of life in patients with advanced cancer

Improve menet	spirit	appetite	Physical strrngth enhance strength enhance	General improve ment	Body weight increase	Sleep inprovee ment	activity capacity improvement and restriced relief	Self-care Walking activities as usual	Return to work Engaged in light body Working
Cases	4071	3986	2450	479	2938	1005	1038	3220	479
(%)	95.2	93.2	57.3	11.2	68.7	23.5	24.3	75.3	11.2

(2) For 84 patients with solid tumors and 56 patients with metastatic supraclavicular lymph nodes, get better results through using oral XZ-C series and external application of XZ-C3 anti-cancer light firming cream. See the table below.

Changes of 84 cases of solid tumors and 56 cases of metastatic nodules after XZ-C cream

	Solid tumor lumps				Cervical supraclavicular lymphadenopathy			
	Disappear	Reduce 1/2	Turn soft	No change	Disappear	Reduce 1/2	Turn soft	No change
Case	12	28	32	12	12	22	14	8
(%)	14.2	33.3	38.0	14.2	21.4	39.2	25.0	14.2
Total efficiency(%)	85.7				85.7			

Analgesic condition after oral administration of XZ-C and external XZ-C anti-cancer analgesic cream in 298 patients

Clinical manifestation	Pain			
	Mild relief	Obvious relief	Disappearance	No effect
Case	52	139	93	14
(%)	17.3	46.8	31.2	4.7
Total effective rate(%)	95.3%			

（十五）15

Immunomodulatory pharmacology of XZ-C immunomodulation anticancer Chinese medication

Compared Western medicine immunopharmacology with traditional Chinese medicine immunopharmacology, each has its own characteristics and advantages. Chinese medication has accumulated a large number of prescriptions through long-term clinical experience with regulating and controlling the body's immune function, especially the beneficial Chinese medication(Replenishment class) which has the effect of regulating and controlling immune activity.

Traditional Chinese medications, whether single-agent or prescription, have multiple active ingredients, unlike Western medications (synthetic drugs) which are single-structured substances. The role of traditional Chinese medicine is multifaceted. In addition to regulating immune function, it has a certain effect on the overall of each functional system.

The main role of XZ-C traditional Chinese medicine immunomodulator in regulating cellular immunity (Cellular immunity) regulates various immune cell-mediated immune responses, including cytokines or lymphokines, and the main function of traditional Chinese medicine immunomodulatory function works on stem cell immunity, such as the thymus, gonads and lymphatic system and T, B cells and various cytokines.

The ancient Chinese medication has the concept of righteousness without weekness or virtual and evil without entering(evil cannot invade) , and constitutes the theoretical component of Chinese medicine. Its essence is to maintain the overall functional balance and enhance disease resistance. Its main role is to enhance the body's immune function. In fact, the tonicmedications (Replenishing drugs) is based on immunopharmacology. Immunopharmacology is a new and emerging marginal discipline that serves as a bridge between pharmacology and immunology. The XZ-C immunomodulator traditional Chinese medication has obvious immune promoting effect.

(十六)16

The indications and application ranges of XZ-C$_{1-10}$ immunomodulation Chinese medication anti-cancer metastasis and recurrence clinical applications

1. a variety of distant metastatic cancer, such as liver metastases, lung metastases, bone metastases, brain metastases, abdominal lymph node metastasis, mediastinal lymph node metastasis, cancerous pleural effusion, cancerous ascites, can come to Wuchang Shuguang oncology clinics for using XZ-C immunomodulation anti-metastatic treatment to stop anti-metastatic steps, and to intervene and block the cancer cells during the metastasis to prolong life.

2. after various radiotherapy and chemotherapy to complete the course of treatment, it should continue to the clinic to take XZ-C1-4 immune control Chinese medicine, in order to consolidate long-term efficacy and prevent recurrence.

3. in the process of radiotherapy and chemotherapy, if the reaction is serious and can not continue, you can come to the Twilight Oncology Clinic and continue to use XZ-C immunomodulation therapy to resist metastasis and recurrence.

4. in the elderly or weekly or infirm patients with other diseases can not be placed, chemotherapy, can come to the Twilight oncology specialist clinic for using XZ-C immunomodulation anti-metastasis and ant-recurrence treatment.

5. The cancer patients who have surgical exploration and the cancer can not cut down, can come to the Twilight oncology specialist outpatient for XZ-C immunomodulation treatment.

6. after palliative surgery, the patient can come to the Twilight oncology specialist clinic for XZ-C immunomodulation anti-metastatic treatment.

7. after a variety of cancer radical surgery, the patient can continue to take XZ-C immune control and regulation anti-cancer Chinese medication to stopm the anti-metastasis, recurrence, in order to improve long-term efficacy.

(十七)17

Study on XZ-C immunomodulation of anticancer traditional Chinese medicine

Table of Contents

I.   *Overview*

II.   *Second, the experimental research and clinical validation work has been carried out*

III.   *Third, the immunopharmacology of XZ-C immunomodulation of traditional Chinese medicine*

IV.   *Fourth, the pharmacodynamics study of XZ-C immunomodulation anti-cancer Chinese medicine*

V.   *The Study on cytokines induced by XZ-C4 anticancer Chinese medication*

VI.   *Sixth. The toxicology research of XZ-C immunomodulation anticancer Chinese medication*

VII.   *Seventh. Regarding Active ingredients of XZ-C immunomodulation anticancer Chinese medication*

VIII.   *Eighth, The principle of XZ-C drug groups*

IX.   *Nineth. Regarding The role of the immune function of the XZ-C immune regulation and control anti-cancer Chinese medications at the molecular level*

X.   *Tenth. The anti-tumor components of XZ-C immunomodulation anti-cancer Chinese medication : structural formula, existing location or site, anti-tumor effect*

XI.   *Evelenth. The Source background and the course of the completion of the project (the tortured process)*

XII.   *Twelve, how can we get out of the squat*

(十八)18

A. **The Partial Cases List of cancer treatment with XZ-C immunomodulation anticancer Chinese medications**

Table of Contents

1. *XZ-C immunomodulation anti-cancer Chinese medicine treatment of partial cases of liver cancer (Case 1 - Case 189)*
2. *XZ-C immunomodulation anticancer Chinese medicine treatment of pancreatic cancer partial cases list (Case 190 - Case 218)*
3. *XZ-C immune regulation anti-cancer Chinese medicine treatment of gastric cancer partial cases list (Case 219 - Case 288)*
4. *XZ-C immune regulation anti-cancer Chinese medicine treatment of some cases of lung cancer (Case 359 - Case 446)*
5. *XZ-C immune regulation anti-cancer Chinese medicine treatment of esophageal cancer partial cases list (Case 447 - Case 481)*
6. *XZ-C immunomodulation anti-cancer Chinese medicine treatment of partial cases of breast cancer (Case 447 - Case 481)*
7. *XZ-C immunomodulation anti-cancer Chinese medicine treatment of some cases of rectal cancer and rectal cancer (case 482 - case 649)*
8. *XZ-C immunomodulation anticancer Chinese medicine for the treatment of cholangiocarcinoma in some cases (case 650 - case 679)Anti-cancer, anti-cancer metastasis research, scientific and technological innovation, scientific research results series*

250

B. **Some typical cases of XZ-C immunomodulation of anticancer traditional Chinese medications in the treatment of malignant tumors**

Table of Contents

1. *Some typical cases of treating liver cancer*
2. *Some typical cases of postoperative adjuvant treatment for pancreatic cancer*
3. *Some typical cases of postoperative adjuvant therapy for gastric cancer*
4. *Some typical cases of postoperative adjuvant treatment for lung cancer*
5. *Some typical cases of postoperative adjuvant therapy for esophageal cancer*
6. *Some typical cases of postoperative adjuvant therapy for breast cancer*
7. *some typical cases of postoperative adjuvant treatment of colorectal cancer*
8. *Some typical cases of postoperative adjuvant therapy for gallbladder cancer*
9. *Some typical cases of postoperative adjuvant therapy for kidney cancer and bladder cancer*
10. *Some typical cases of postoperative adjuvant therapy such as thyroid cancer and retroperitoneal tumor*
11. *Some typical cases of non-Hodgkin's lymphoma treatment*
12. *chemotherapy + XZ-C Chinese medicine treatment of acute lymphoblastic leukemia typical cases*
13. *Some typical cases of ovarian cancer and cervical cancer treatment*

Strive to take the road of innovation in China's characteristic anti-cancer metastasis

Take the road of modernization of traditional Chinese medications, promote the integration of Chinese and Western medicine at the molecular level, and integrate with the modernization of international medicine.

19

The formation of the theoretical system of XZ-C treatment

In the book "New Concepts and New Methods of Cancer Treatment", Professor Xu Ze used 30 years of self-reliance and hard work to complete the basic and clinical research of the "Eighth Five-Year Plan" of the National Science and Technology Commission. Nearly 100 research papers summarizing a series of scientific research results were published in the form of the new books.

This book has formed the theoretical system of XZ-C cancer treatment, which is the clinical basis and experimental basis for cancer treatment and has undergone the clinical application observation and verification.

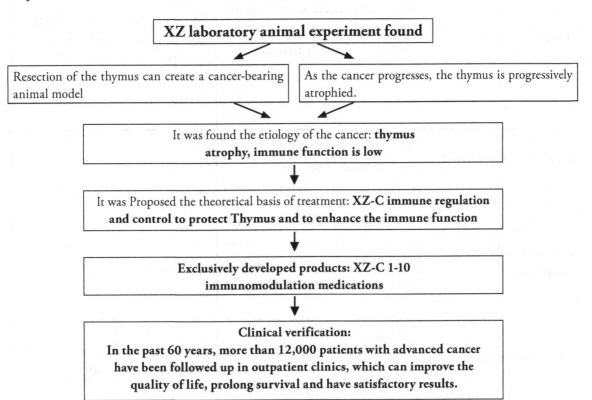

XZ laboratory animal experiment found

| Resection of the thymus can create a cancer-bearing animal model | As the cancer progresses, the thymus is progressively atrophied. |

It was found the etiology of the cancer: **thymus atrophy, immune function is low**

It was Proposed the theoretical basis of treatment: **XZ-C immune regulation and control to protect Thymus and to enhance the immune function**

Exclusively developed products: XZ-C 1-10 immunomodulation medications

Clinical verification:
In the past 60 years, more than 12,000 patients with advanced cancer have been followed up in outpatient clinics, which can improve the quality of life, prolong survival and have satisfactory results.

XZ-C theoretical system for cancer treatment
(XZ-C)(XU ZE-China)(China-Xu Ze)

20

The book proposed XZ-C new concept cancer therapy, which was analyzed and compared with traditional therapy, and analyzed by table:

	XZ new concept of cancer therapy	Traditional chemotherapy and radiotherapy cancer therapy
Theoretical basis	The new concept says: Cure or Healing should be regulated and control rather than killed	The traditional concept holds or says: he goal of treatment must be to kill cancer cells
Etiology, pathogenesis	Thymus atrophy Low immune function	(——)
The theoretical basis and experimental basis of treatment	Immune regulation and control ; Protection of Thymus and Increase of immune function	(——)
Treatment principles	To Establish a comprehensive view of treatment.	Single target killing cancer cells and One-sided treatment

Treatment mode	Full treatment: surgery + biology immune regulation and control Short-course treatment: radiotherapy, chemotherapy Not long term and do not overdose	Chemotherapy + radiotherapy Or release + chemotherapy Or radiotherapy +chemotherapy synchronize
Medication therapy	XZ-C 1-10 immune regulation and control Modernization of traditional Chinese medicine and the combination of Chinese and Western medications at the molecular level	Cytotoxic drugs (both killing cancer cells and killing normal proliferating cells)
Complications, side effects	no	Toxic side effects, some have serious toxic side effects
Efficacy	Improve quality of life and prolong survival	Relieve for a few months, and may relapse
Medical expenses	Significantly reduced medical expenses	Medical expenses are large, nearly 100 billion yuan per year in China
prospect	Walked on a new way of combining immune control with Chinese and Western medicine and cancer treatment	The effect is relieved, still stagnation

Printed in the United States
By Bookmasters